Where do Daddies Come From?

A Pregnancy Bible for Men

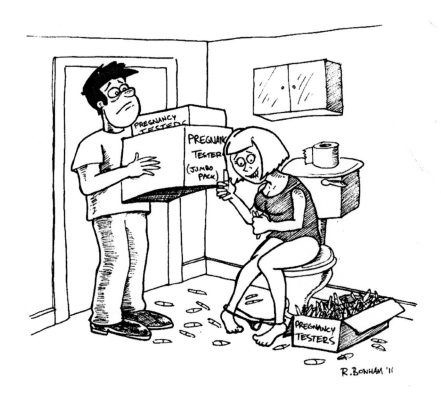

R. BONHAM '11

Steve Cummins

GLASNEVIN
PUBLISHING

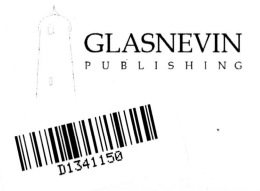

Where do Daddies Come From?
A Pregnancy Bible for Men

Steve Cummins

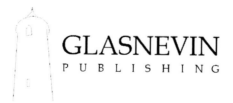

GLASNEVIN PUBLISHING

First published in 2011 by

Glasnevin Publishing
16 Griffith Parade
Glasnevin
Dublin 11
Ireland

www.glasnevinpublishing.com

A CIP catalogue record for this book is available from the British Library

ISBN: 978-1-9086890-0-9

This book is dedicated to my beautiful wife Nuala,

Also

To Leon and Sam.

The best parts of me.

CONTENTS

Chapter 5: Strippers, Midwives & Cops

Chapter 6: Pethedine and Poop

Chapter 7: Tit Nazis and Tears

Chapter 8: Blue Balls and Benny Hill

Disclaimer

The author and the publisher are not liable or responsible to any person or entity for any damage caused or alleged to be caused directly or indirectly by the information contained in this book.

Note from the Author

I am not a gynaecologist. I am not a nurse, midwife or doctor. I have never had any medical training whatsoever except a first aid course where I arrived with a force five hangover and nearly threw up in the CPR dummy. I claim no special medical knowledge whatsoever. I am a comedian and writer who also happens to be a loving husband and dad. I would describe my research techniques as sketchy at best. Most of my information is internet based and I was pretty half assed in double checking my facts. What I'm getting at here is that I do not claim to be any kind of expert. This book is a mixture of facts, opinion and gutter humour. It's not meant to be taken too seriously. I'm bound to have made mistakes along the way so take everything I say with a grain or two of salt. Okay, enough sugar coating it. Don't sue me. That's all I care about. I don't want some moron who takes some joke in this book seriously, who then goes and fires his wife from a catapult or something, to decide that the funny book made him do it and go hire a lawyer. So remember if you sue an author the terrorists win. (That should keep the crazies in line)

Steve Cummins, October 2011

ABOUT THE AUTHOR

Steve Cummins is a comedian, broadcaster and writer. Before this incarnation he worked with juvenile offenders in the U.K. Ireland and the U.S.A. He has appeared on the BBC, RTE, Channel 4 and TG4. Steve is a headliner in every major comedy club in Ireland and regularly performs abroad. Steve is a regular contributor to nearly every major radio station. He has written for three television projects and created, wrote and presented the comedy panel show; "What Were We Thinking?" for the national broadcaster 2FM, which aired in January 2011.

He is married to the long suffering Nuala and has two beautiful boys, Leon aged eight and Sam aged three. He lives by the sea in Rush Co. Dublin.

ACKNOWLEDGEMENTS

There are very few people to thank as I wrote this book all by myself. Screw it. Now that I think about it you should be thanking me. I bust my ass writing this.

Okay then, with as much bad grace as possible I'd like to thank the following people without whom this book would still have been written but it might have been ever so slightly different.

To Robbie Bonham without whose amazing cartoons this book would be a least eight pages shorter.

To Matthew Collins who helped come up with the title for this book. I still wish I'd called it "It's not Uteryou it's Uterus" but what do I know? I'm just the talent.

To Bryan from Glasnevin Publishing who not only gave me a book deal and then had the good sense to just let me get on with it but he laughed at my act too.

To Peter O'Mahony and Eoin Byrne whose input really taught me to never ask for advice.

To all the dads who freely gave five minutes of their lives to fill out a questionnaire and offer me their invaluable wisdom. Now your name is in print. Lucky bastards.

To my beautiful wife Nuala who never believed this book would get published…Fuck you honey, fuck you.

Finally to my two amazing, beautiful boys Leon and Sam. If this book is a bestseller it still doesn't make up for all the sleep I've lost.

INTRODUCTION

Well you did it. Whether you meant to or not is immaterial. You went and knocked her up. If you meant to do it and it was planned and all, congratulations, you are about to enter an amazing chapter in your life. If you did it by accident and it was about as planned as your stag party in Afghanistan, commiserations, you are about to enter an amazing chapter in your life. Either way, here is your bible. I promise you I will be able to answer a lot of your questions about pregnancy, labour and the first few weeks of life for the little monster, (Or monsters, you never thought about twins did you?). If the only question you have is, "Is it my baby?" I can't answer that. Try Jerry Springer and you might want to examine your relationship. Just a suggestion.

What are my qualifications I hear you cry? Who am I to be offering so much tongue-in-cheek yet somehow infinitely wise advice? Well, I have no qualifications save being the father of two strong, beautiful boys. One of whom came as a bigger shock than George W getting elected to a second term while the other was more planned than Stalin's first five years in power. One was an emergency caesarean while the other was pushed out in a shower of urine and expletives (mostly from me I might add).

I am a professional comedian and really good at it. This has had the added benefits of my having taken care of my boys since my wife finished maternity leave because I work mostly at night (Yes, I am a yummy mummy). Add to that the fact that I will not be taking too much of this book seriously. Don't worry, you will learn lots but that doesn't mean that you can't have a laugh while you do so. Pregnancy and babies are an amazing experience and a huge challenge at the same time. You are about to be given an incredible gift, one you will love in a way you heretofore never thought possible. You are also going to feel left out, alienated, confused, terrified and grossed out. Horny too, but what else is new.

While everyone accepts and makes allowances for the mother, no one ever thinks of the father (except maybe your friends but they're just going to take the piss). This is not going to change so you'd better start getting used to it. Always remember that she is the one whose body is going to go through massive physiological changes and for dessert go through massive physical trauma. The best description I have ever heard to try to get men to understand the pain of childbirth is "Imagine shitting a microwave". It's crude but it makes me wince every time I think of it - I think it's imagining the corners. Which would you prefer: feeling left out, or pushing out a major kitchen appliance? I thought so.

Now, as I said, get used to feeling at best, like a useless, spare wheel whose opinion is valued about as much as Zimbabwean currency or at worst, as the enemy. Not just from her but from any woman who has ever experienced it. That's what this book is for. It's there to hold your hand, soothe your fevered brow and most importantly, to give you a place where you can vent your feelings of rage. And have a bit of a sulk at times too. This is a book for men.

By all means read her the odd excerpt (I even put in a few paragraphs that keep her sweet for this very reason) but for the love of God don't let her get her hands on it. Guard this book as you would your porn. Coincidentally, your porn will take on new importance to help you get through the; tender boobs, morning sickness, "I hate my body" lean spells as well. Hide it well. We all have a porn stash hidden better than Osama Bin Laden so just keep it there and sneak it into the bathroom when you need it. Remember when they found Bin Laden? He apparently was found with a huge stash of porn – what an amateur! The Navy S.E.A.L.s may find me but they would never find my porn. No way.

This book is going to be divided into neat little chapters. Each one takes about the same time to read as the average male bowel movement so it's digestible in easy form if you'll forgive the pun. Take it into the loo with you when its time to bake some brownies and you should have it finished in about a fortnight. If it takes longer to finish than six weeks you are either too dumb to grasp even simple concepts or you have Irritable Bowel Syndrome. If it's the former I have put some colouring-in at the back of the book just for you. See, it's a foetus. If it's the latter don't lend this book to anyone. Burn it when you're done and don't ever shake my hand if we meet.

Despite my immature attitude there is actually a serious element to this book. I truly believe that most men would like to take a more active role in the pregnancy but lack of knowledge is really holding them back. The professionals are too concerned with the woman to be able to, or even want to, teach you so most men end up spending the pregnancy wondering what the hell happened to the woman they love and spending the birth standing around trying not to puke or giggle. I was less than useless during my wife's first pregnancy and spent my time during the labour trying to sneak sly whiffs of the Gas & Air (Why should she have all the fun?) while jumping out of the way whenever anyone barked at me. When it came to my second son I was older, more experienced and much more aware of what my wife needed/wanted. I was better prepared for the insanity that was her pregnancy and way better equipped to help in the labour ward. I got to spend the time they were stitching up my wife relishing the mountain of praise being heaped on me by all the midwives. It was the cries of "if there was more men like you" etc that gave me the idea for this book. Don't get me wrong, I love praise and will take it from any corner regardless of how false it is, but in this case I knew I'd deserved it. If I had been as knowledgeable for my first son as I was for my second one I would have been a huge help to my wife. This book will help you to help her and even help yourself (How disgustingly New Age is that last sentence?). Let's try that again. This book contains answers and opinions that I have learned, picked up and made up over the course of two pregnancies. There are also some quotes from fathers from all walks of life from comedians and broadcasters to Taekwondo masters and butchers. These will help to show you that you're not alone. Other men felt the exact same feelings you're going through right now. They got through it and so will you.

I promise only one thing to you. This book will help. It will make you laugh, it will teach you a lot and it will show you that pretty much whatever you're feeling is normal and that you'll cope. It will help you be a better man to her during this tumultuous time and it will stop you from loading up the car with clothes and CD's and driving off into the sunset. Okay, I promise only six things. If you bought this book for yourself: well done in being proactive. If it was bought for you by a friend: thank them and if they are that nice you can probably hit them up for babysitting later. If this was bought for you by the woman in your life then she's noticed you haven't a clue or she's trying to get you to show some interest in the whole thing. Finally, if you rented this book from the library I haven't made a penny so, screw you cheapskate.

So, to everyone without a library card; enjoy the book and good luck. You're going to need it.

Chapter 1

The Booby Fairy Cometh

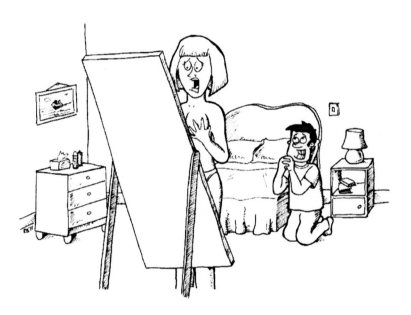

"I swear I think my boobs are getting bigger."

In the Beginning…..

How long does pregnancy last? Nine months, right? Wrong. Its forty weeks or roughly 266 days or 6384 hours or 383,040 minutes or 22,982,400 seconds of fun, fun, fun (Can you tell I own a calculator?). Imagine that - just under twenty three million seconds. Well that should just fly by. So whenever your beloved is finding the whole pregnancy difficult just tell her to subtract the number of seconds she's been pregnant from 23 million and she'll see how time is racing by. Don't worry, she'll be delighted. Pregnant women love maths. Why do you think they're always calculating? Due dates, ovulation schedules, counting contractions, how many drinks you've had, even adding up all the weight they've put on. So, when the going gets tough just toss her a calculator (imagine what she'd do to you with a pencil…yikes) and watch her happy face light up.

The good news is that if you're reading this you're probably at least a few months in so you can knock off a few million already. See: you're half way there. I honestly don't know where the nine month figure came from. Some say that women use a special secret calendar for all things. Time runs differently for women. They have a completely different system than men. We sit and listen to a woman talk about her day for seven hours she feels we've only been chatting for twenty seconds. We've been performing sexual gymnastics for hours yet she seems to feel like it was just a few minutes. Sure the alarm clock's red glow backs her up but I've never trusted technology.

Stevie's month by month guide to the creature inside her: 1st month

The creature is smaller then a grain of rice and looks a hell of a lot more like a tadpole than a human. Freaky fact: It has a tail! A tail for Christ's sake. This is probably why they don't take scan pictures of it yet. Imagine showing that to your co-workers.

The actual mathematicians out there are probably thinking that if we are dealing with four week months not calendar months then the ten month figure is completely accurate. Well, screw you for being so pedantic. Why are you even reading this book? There's no way you even slept with a girl let alone got one pregnant - unless they were attracted to your calculating ability. That must be it. Damn you nerds, you win again.

Anyway, it doesn't really matter whether you say nine months or ten because at the end of the day neither of you will have much say in when it decides to come out. Lets just keep it simple and all agree to say its 23 million seconds and let that be an end to it. Before we can move on however I feel we need to decide on a few ground rules.

First of all, this book will be peppered with swear words. That's okay because they are just words and as we all know, words can never hurt you. That is, unless of course you work in the finance industry. Then here's a word that'll ruin your day…redundancy. Screw you. I've been getting threatening letters from the banks for years. It's my turn now. Here's a tip: if you want a bit of fun, go into your local bank branch with a copy of the latest share prices, queue for three hours and when you eventually get to the counter show the cashier how badly their bank is doing and ask them if they want a loan. You may think that's cruel and very childish but from now on you'll have to take little pleasures wherever you can get them.

Back to the swear words. If for some insane reason you have a problem with bad language then you'd better man up and fast. It doesn't matter how demur your lady is, when she starts pushing she'll teach you swear words you never knew existed. I don't think Mother Teresa ever gave birth but if she did I bet the expression "I'll shove my motherfucking sandals up your motherfucking arse" was bandied about. There are three reasons that this book has swearing in it.
1. We're men. It's expected.
2. It helps. Believe me.
3. To answer Mr. O'Brien, my teacher in fourth class, Yes, I do think it's big and clever.

Okay, so if all the sensitive souls, the easily offended and the pedantic have left we can continue. Swearing stays. Fuck yeah.

The second thing we need to sort out is what term we're going to use for our pregnant angel (don't worry; there's no way we're calling her that). Not everyone is married so we can't use wife or missus. We're not in a seventies British sitcom so we can't use 'er indoors. We can't use the terms lover or special lady because we're not creepy serial killers. You get the idea. I think we should use the terms "Her" and "She". We'll capitalise them just to make our special lady feel special.

Wait, I never said special lady. I meant woman. Please don't dig up my patio.

Her and She are ideal for two reasons. Firstly I think I can make a pretty broad assumption here that your She is a woman. I'm no doctor but I'm pretty sure She needs to be one in order to be pregnant. Secondly, if you put the two words together they sound like Hershey which is a type of chocolate - something which could save your life one day soon. Always have a few treats in your pocket to appease Her: Sugar lumps, fun size chocolate bars, legs of lamb. You get the idea. Also, if you get bored you can scour the book counting the number of times I forgot to capitalise Her and she (there's one to get you started). After that maybe you can go and count the number of birds that fly past your house in a given day. I bet you're the sort of person who points out mistakes when people have just finished wallpapering a room. In short, you're a douche.

The third and final ground rule is this. I am making the assumption that you love and care for Her. While I will be regularly making fun of and at times railing against Her, this book is meant to be here to help both of you. To offer advice, tips and tricks to help you get through this wild time while also giving you the skills for helping Her as much as possible. So, if you were thinking why not just call Her "the bitch who ruined my life" then perhaps you should set the book down slowly and walk away.

Okay, ground rules aside it's time to get this party started. Never has the term party been so inappropriately used (well except maybe the Nazi party but I'm not touching that with a barge pole). Let's face it: you're shitting yourself and if you're not you should be. A baby is for life, not just for Christmas. You can't just leave food out for it and let it crap in the neighbour's garden. You have just been handed a massive responsibility. Forget your job, your mortgage, even your marriage. This is the most serious long term commitment there is. You can always quit your job, sell your house or divorce your wife but this will always be your child. Your blood, your responsibility, always and forever. Amen. It's up to you to keep it safe, raise it, teach it, love it, discipline it, feed it, clothe it, bathe it, nurture it and do God alone knows what else for it. You and only you have the hugest role in this child's life. You will be its father. Stop a moment, seriously, put down the book for a second and take a moment to get your head around that. I'll wait.

Thank God you're back. You took ages. How huge is that? You. A father. A Dad. You can't be a Dad. It's too soon. You're not ready. Well guess what Daddio? You're never ready to be a father. It just happens. Your father wasn't ready, his father before him wasn't ready. I don't know about his father before that, I ran out of funding in my research. The point is that the old cliché about there being no manual for parenthood is rubbish. There are millions of them. You can find books to tell you how to do everything from changing nappies to deciding which mood suppressant to give them when they're a bit attention deficit. However there is no manual for being a father.

That word is one of the biggest in the world. Think about your own father. Whether he was loving and attentive or about as involved in rearing you as Odysseus (Greek mythology, left home for twenty years, son resented it and eventually killed him. Talk about a laboured metaphor) either way he had a fundamental role in creating the man you are today. Even an absent father can be a role model. He may teach his son that family isn't important and that it's okay to walk away from your responsibilities or his absence might teach you the importance of having a positive male role model in your life.

What if I am a Bad Father?

Everyone starts out as a bad father, just as there is no magically perfect first time mother. We all have to wing it in the beginning. You arrive home from hospital with a tiny helpless creature and have no idea what to do with it. The simple equation is this: if you love your child more than yourself (and you will) then you're going to be a great father. Unless you're shite.

I was born without a father. Or to be more precise, he either left around the time I was born or he died the day I was born in a car crash on the way to see me in the hospital. Forgive the ambiguity but details were always a little hazy. All that's important is that I grew up without a father. So I looked for one. I don't mean I wandered the streets eyeing up potential daddies to bring home to my abandoned/widowed mother. I mean I got my daddy lessons from TV. That really wasn't such a bad thing. TV in the seventies and eighties was black and white. I don't mean the sets themselves, I mean the content. Good guys were always good. Bad guys were always bad and fathers always loved their kids and tried to do the very best by them. I wanted to be the hero in the white hat. I grew up with phrases like "A man's gotta do what a man's gotta do" and "You've got to look out for the little guy" and "How do they get the figs into the fig rolls?" Okay, the last one not so much but you get the idea. Today's TV and movie stars all have feet of clay and suffer from crises of conscience daily. Sure, the hero saves the day but he's a recovering alcoholic who's ex wife won't speak to him and whose kids are afraid of him at best and ambivalent towards him at worst.

Think of the TV dads of the eighties. Heathcliffe Huxtable in The Cosby show, Stephen Keaton in Family Ties, Crazy Adolph in Mein Father Der Fuhrer. Maybe I dreamed the last one but the point is those dads didn't have feet of clay. They loved their kids and managed to solve all their problems in less than half an hour. Here's my list of how a TV dad acted.
- TV dads always wore loud jumpers.
- TV dads always made time to listen to their kids.
- TV dads always made it home on time to eat with their kids.
- TV dads never swore.
- TV dads didn't hit their kids.
- TV dads always had the right answer.
- TV dads always had a hot wife.

I look over this list and I see just how much they moulded me.
- I have terrible dress sense.
- I try to listen to my kids although sometimes they bore the piss out of me. (I don't care what the fuck Barney thinks about marching).
- I work from home or at night so I don't exactly have to brave the commute.

6

- Okay, nobody's fucking perfect.
- I have never hit my kids although I would have no hesitation beating the crap out of someone else's.
- Of course I have all the right answers. I'm a man.
- Smoking hot. Women love a guy with a sense of humour, thank Christ.

Whether my father was a deadbeat dad or at the very least a bad driver I managed to avoid both of those fates (Only two points on my licence) and instead I grew up with an old fashioned idea of how a father should be. It doesn't make me perfect by any means but no one is. You won't be a perfect father no matter how hard you try. If you love your child, and you will, believe me, then all you have to do is what's right.

Easy? Of course not. But here's the important bit. Try your best, love your child and enjoy the ride. At the end of the day your kids will blame you for all their hang ups and neuroses anyway so you might as well chill the fuck out.

Stevie's month by month guide to the creature inside her: 2nd month

Good news, the tail is gone. Ratbaby is no more. It's now developing arms and legs, even fingers and toes. It's around an inch long now. Freaky fact, it has eyes but its eyelids are sealed shut like some horror movie extra.

Time to Man Up

Okay. Here we go. No more screwing around. It's time to step up to the plate. Here we go. Okay. This is it. Okay. Here we go. No more procrastination. See where I'm going with this?

You've got less than nine months dude. You don't have time for your usual, the world will end/I'll win the lottery, get out clauses. By the way the world might end or you may even win the lottery. I have a theory that I always throw at those dicks who like to quote you the odds of winning the lottery when they hear that

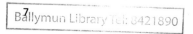

you do it. I always tell them that it's not 14 million to 1 or whatever. I tell them that your odds of winning the lottery are fifty/fifty. Either you will or you won't. Flawless logic!

Stephen Hawking couldn't talk his way around that one. It's amazing I ever got this book finished really. See? There I go again. Procrastinating, but this time there's a point to it. The time for procrastination is past. That was your last little bit of it - at least where this book is concerned. There's a baby in there and it's coming out sooner rather than later so you need to get with the programme. Speaking of programmes, I love a good sitcom. Sure, Friends is a bit dated today but when it was current...Damn it! The baby! Got it. Seriously, that was the last time.

I don't know what stage in the game you're reading this but I'll assume it's early on. If you're frantically flicking through this while shoving a baby back in with your foot then it's probably a bit too late for you. Take your foot off the baby and go help your wife with pushing. Out, not in. So, for the rest of you, the normal ones, the ride has begun. Please keep your arms in the car at all times and please remember that it was keeping something inside for too long got you in this mess in the first place.

She's pregnant. You did it. Just accept it. Now you feel either one of two ways:
1. You're delighted and a bit scared but ultimately excited at the prospect of being a father. You acknowledge that it's going to be difficult initially but so rewarding that all the sleepless nights and worry are far outweighed by the long term joy that fatherhood is.
2. Your life is over.
If you are from the latter camp don't worry this is entirely normal and kind of true too. If, however you fall into the first category then you are a weirdo. Seriously, long term joy? Jesus, where did you come up with that? Drop this book and go buy something from the Women's Interest section. Douche.

Sorry about that. Where were we? Oh yeah, your life is over. I'd love to tell you something different but I can't. Your life as you knew it is essentially over. Let's start off small. You will never go to the cinema to see anything but a kid's movie ever again. This is for the simple reason that if your babysitter's hourly rate is more than you make in a day then you're going drinking. There's no way you're shelling out all that money to go see a romcom, believe me. Even if you don't drink now: give it time. A few months of parenthood and you'll both drink like its St. Patricks Day every chance you get. If you are a drinker: guess what? Spontaneous drinking is no longer an option. Remember all those Sunday afternoon pub lunches that led on to week long binges. Well, no more. Remember when you'd leave work at eleven thirty and wake up in a Guatemalan prison four days later? Wave bye-bye to those. One of you will have to get up with the baby. Even when they're sleeping the night through it still means you'll probably be up before six. Now imagine that with a force ten hangover. Oh dear God. Forget water boarding. If you want to get a terrorist to talk just make him change a shitty nappy that smells like cat food while suffering through a five tequila hangover. Oh, the humanity.

The only way you can successfully get pissed occasionally is through give and take. Who gets to drink becomes a more delicate negotiation than the last UN charter. My personal favourite was the "I'll drive there and you can drive back" technique. This works well during pregnancy and if there's breastfeeding on the cards - for the baby, not you. Pervert! Eventually however she'll see through this and you'll need to come up with a strategy.

Speaking of breastfeeding, you might as well give it a go! What with expressing, posseting (that's baby milk puke to you and me), leakage and God knows what else you're going to become contaminated at some stage so you might as well take charge of how it happens. I personally recommend having a taste of some expressed milk. Going straight to the well might be creepy for both of you. Or worse still, creepy for just one of you. Try it. It tastes weirdly sweet and I guarantee you'll never try it again. This is why I recommend you have an open beer at the ready. Or twelve open beers - whatever it takes.

If you're formula feeding there's no point in tasting it. It's commonly used to cut cocaine with so you've probably tasted it already. So just go buy some cocaine. That's why I recommend an open beer at the ready. Or twelve open beers, a bottle of vodka and a shotgun. Damn it. It's Guatemala all over again. Okay, no coke alright? Maybe that's why they say breast is best.

Seriously though, I know I said your life as you know it is over, and it is, but it is entering a new and genuinely wonderful phase. I will talk more about going out, breast milk and even cocaine as the book progresses. I am going to be making fun of you around every corner but I promise you it comes from a good place. As I said, I know you're freaked out but don't be scared. Take my hand in a completely heterosexual way and come with me on the most amazing journey of your life. How new age and wanky was that last sentence?

How did you react on being told that you were about to become a father?

After being told I spent rest of the day in A&E. After hearing "I'm pregnant" I passed out, hit my head off an open oven door and got 14 stitches in the side of my head.

Paraic, Butcher

Ch ch ch ch changes…

Okay, the woman you adore is going to go through some changes, actually, lots of changes and all of them will affect you. Some are great, others are awful. First of all, let's look at the physiological changes. I want to start on a positive note. One morning in or around the third month something wonderful is going to happen. Your angel will get out of bed and you'll notice something wonderful. At some time in the night The Booby Fairy will have visited and turned your missus into a porn star. No, not all pouty and pizza guy obsessed, her boobs will have grown at an alarming rate.
- If she was small before she is now big.
- If she was big before she is now enormous.
- If she was enormous before, buy a crash helmet and best of luck.

The Booby Fairy is, of course, easily explained by doctors as the body preparing itself for feeding of the new born infant. I think the real truth is that God sends him as some sort of reward to you for not killing the hormonal psychopath who now shares your bed. Whatever the truth is you are now spending time with a woman you clearly love and respect and she is now in possession of a new body. Make the most of this. Get to know the new boobies, play with them, enjoy them while you can because pretty soon they will be too tender to touch and when that passes there is a good chance that you'll no longer have sole access to them. However for the moment, all is rosy in the garden. She has a tidy wee bump to stroke and you have new boobies to do likewise.

Being pregnant is new and exciting for her and labour is far enough away to be just an occasional anxiety which has been filed away in that computer like brain of hers under "I" for "I'll deal with that later". Somewhere between "I can't believe he said that to my mother" and "I'll tell him all about that when I get home". One thing which shocked the hell out of me was that my wife's nipples changed colour. I don't mean like a traffic light, red, amber, green - I mean they got darker, much darker. I know, who expects that to happen? It wasn't a big deal but I wasn't expecting it either. I kept waiting for them to start pointing in different directions but thankfully that doesn't happen - except maybe in zero gravity but unless she is an astronaut or works testing roller coasters I don't see that happening.

Oh, and her belly button can also go from an innie to an outie. I have to tell you, that freaks you out when you first notice it. It makes you think that the baby is trying to push itself out like in the movie Alien. It's totally normal. All the changes are normal but that doesn't make it any less weird for either of you. Remember that she will be as freaked out as you are. In fact, she'll probably be even more so. You are only observing these changes, she has to live them. Every single day.

Enough of the physical, lets get to the meat and potatoes of this whole pregnancy lark. There is something you need to know about the pregnant one. The woman you loved is gone! The rational, happy, loving woman who makes your heart flutter whenever you see her unexpectedly has left for the time being. Where once your heart used to soar with love and excitement it will now grow icy cold as you hear her come through the front door. Living with a pregnant woman is like living with a multiple personality schizophrenic. Not the fun kind of multiple personality schizophrenic. You know the type: one day thinks they're Napoleon the next day they are baking you a cake. No,

I'm talking about the "Favah beans and a nice Chianti" type of one: the type who keeps buying pets but never any pet food - if you know what I mean.

She's nuts dude. That's what I'm trying to tell you.

Sure, the woman you love is in there and she even comes out occasionally but she now shares the space with the hormonal equivalent of the seven dwarves.

1. Happy
2. Grumpy
3. Sleepy
4. Weepy
5. Angry
6. Furious
7. Hungry

You honestly never know who's looking at you and believe me you better not make a mistake. Sure Disney made the whole seven dwarves thing look cute but imagine the reality: seven men with a physical disability living together and working in the highly risky world of diamond mining (anyone ever hear of blood diamonds?). Each and every one of these potential warlords, with their own specific mental disorder or allergy (Sneezy, clever huh?). Would you allow your beautiful daughter to shack up with them? Of course not. You'd rather she hooked up with a biker gang or a born again Christian. Remember it's a war so it's vitally important to know your enemy. Let's look at the combatants.

First there's Happy - the rarest of the dwarves. He comes out in those times when the pregnant one is full, rested and is all excited at the thought of having a baby. This is the dwarf to ask favours of. Little things like, "Can I go out with the lads for a quick round of golf?" or "May I please stop sleeping in the shed?" It is advisable for you to get a notary or solicitor to take a record of whatever concessions she makes because most of the other dwarves will try their best to renege on them. Happy is the dwarf who most closely resembles the one you love. Cherish Happy's brief visits. Sometimes, like letters from home to a soldier at war, that's the only thing that gets you through it.

Grumpy is quite a common visitor but needs to be handled carefully as he has been known to hand off to one of the other, more frightening dwarves if provoked. Grumpy is usually best handled with compliments and vast amounts of whatever food Grumpy feels like at that precise time. I say "at that time" because food tastes and fads change almost as fast as moods do, so never, ever choose the food yourself. You are just as likely to end up wearing the meal as eating it.

Sleepy is a very welcome dwarf. Sleepy is there to give you, not her, a chance for some well earned rest from all the anxiety of wondering what her next commands shall be. Sleepy comes at strange times however. Sleepy may decide that seven in the evening is the best time to visit but then might decide to fuck off at three AM and leave one of the other dwarves holding the fort. Basically, Sleepy can't be trusted but like those moments at work when you sneak off to another floor for a sneaky crap, he is to be cherished and like fine weather in April you have no idea how long it will last but you are going around in Speedo's while it does.

Weepy is a very common visitor and while he doesn't stay around for long he must be respected and treated with kid gloves because he is very close friends with Angry and Furious. Two dwarves you really, really don't want to mess with.

Angry and Furious, I have always suspected, are brothers and very close. They are the hormonal equivalent of The Kray twins but much more violent. Where one goes the other is sure to be close behind. These two are worse than all the others combined. When I heard that Lorena Bobbitt had famously hacked off her husband's manhood and thrown it out of the window of her speeding car I was convinced that she must have been pregnant. It turns out she was just insane. Can you imagine how much worse she would have been if she was pregnant? I don't even want to talk about these two for too long as I am still suffering from post traumatic stress. Suffice it to say: you will meet them and no matter how tough you think you are, you'll run and no man will ever judge you for it. Run Forrest, Run.

Hungry is the last of the dwarves and is going to be your constant companion. Pregnant women eat - all the time. It may feel like they are eating for six but for the love of God let them. Hungry is the only dwarf who has the ear and immediate support of all the other dwarves. If you try to deny Hungry anything, hell even if you delay Hungry, Hungry will call all the other dwarves to rain hellfire down upon you.

You may think it's impossible to feel so many emotions all at once and for you and I it is, but not for them. There are other dwarves that I haven't even mentioned here. Some too terrifying to talk about and also my seven dwarves analogy wouldn't have worked. You'll meet them all but to continue with my earlier analogy of the soldier at war - hang in there private, it will end. Maybe not in time for Christmas, but it will end. You'll get to see your gal again and maybe, just maybe, peace will reign.

> ***How did you react on being told that you were about to become a father?***
>
> My wife woke me at six in the morning. She did the test in the bathroom and came running in to tell me. I congratulated her and went back to sleep.
>
> Patrick. Actor & Comedian

Here is a perfect example of living with a pregnant woman. I remember once having a blazing row with my wife as we drove to the Chinese take away. I don't know what it was about. Probably the fact that I would only let her order the left half of the menu as opposed to the whole thing or more than likely the fact that I wasn't breaking the sound barrier to get her to the food. Anyway, I left a screaming dervish in the car while I went to collect our order. As I was paying for it I asked them to throw in a bag of prawn crackers purely on a whim, I honestly don't know why. I reluctantly got back in the car and threw the bag of food to her before she could maul me like some lion in a safari park. Silence descended as she tore open the bag and the next thing a sobbing creature was hugging me and planting wet kisses all over my cheek. You see, to you and I, the prawn crackers were just that. Some crackers covered with mystery prawn flavoured MSG. To her however, they were proof positive that not only did I love her but that I would also be a good provider for the baby. See what I mean?

If anyone else acted like that you'd have them committed and you can only imagine the stress of living from minute to minute not knowing if you are the world's greatest husband or some reincarnation of Hitler.

Top Five Movies She Had Better Not Watch

1. Rosemary's baby
2. Alien
3. The Omen
4. Demon Seed
5. Mamma Mia (Just because it's shit)

How Much is All This Going to Cost?

Holy shit! - babies are expensive, really, really expensive. From the moment you pay for an overpriced stick for Her to pee on to the day when you're in your eighties and they come looking for a loan. That wee bundle of joy will be a greater strain on your finances than a severe cocaine habit. Granted, it's doubtful you'll ever offer to suck the dick of a nappy salesman but you will constantly be hit by expense after expense. By the way, I know there's no such thing as a nappy salesman but the analogy wouldn't work without it so go watch the movie Menace 2 Society and you'll see just how clever that was.

Just for starters you will need;
- Somewhere for it to sleep. I know it would fit in your underpants drawer but seriously, what sort of a start in life is that? You'll need to get a Moses basket which, disappointingly, is not as cool as it sounds. If you drop your baby in a river in this it'll sink like a stone. Trust me on this. The Moses basket is really just for the first few weeks, maybe months, but then you'll need a cot. Basically a mini baby prison with bars and everything. Be sure to search your baby regularly for shanks. Never accept a carton of cigarettes from your baby. If you do you'll forever be its bitch. Mind you, you'll be its bitch regardless of what you do. It craps itself and you run and wipe its ass. Who's the real bitch in this scenario? Not shitty bum that's for sure.

- Clothes - lots and lots and lots of clothes. Babygrows, bodysuits, booties, and that's just the B's. By the time you get to zebra patterned cowboy boots you'll practically be bankrupt. I'm kidding about the boots but what do you bet that someone will read this and start manufacturing them? You heard it here first folks. Soon, when the streets are awash with boot wearing babies and all you can hear is the sound of spurs jingling in crèches all across the land I'll want my cut of the action. You'll back me up in court right? Seriously though, you'll spend a fortune on clothes. Sure people give you loads of clothes after the birth but it's usually newborn sized so by the time the baby is six months old it starts to look like the incredible Hulk after he has changed back into Bruce Banner: all tattered clothes that barely cover the nappy. Some kind friends and relatives will give you their old baby clothes. The truly well meaning will give you bags of clean, well cared for clothes which will save you a fortune. The less well meaning will use you as an informal clothes bank and will unload any old crap they have lying around. Whatever old faded and torn clothes they have cluttering up their home are yours to decorate your baby with. The hilarious thing is these are the ones who'll complain if you don't dress your baby in their dross. Accept all the baby clothes you want but keep them safe because some people expect their clothes back. Nothing tears at the bonds of friendship like two women fighting over baby clothes. It's usually safer to accept clothes only from relatives and the sanest relatives at that. In other words - not hers.

- Nappies. When you stand back and take a look at how much you are going to spend for years on disposable toilets for the world's most accomplished incontinent you'll cry harder than your baby will when they realise they have your genes (I'm talking to you baldy/fatty/pancreatic cancery). Nappies cost a fortune but you'll gladly pay it. The alternative is using terry cloth nappies. These are basically like the little hand towels you steal from hotels. You fold them just right and seal them with a large lethal looking safety pin. The real fun is that you get to keep a load of these steeping in chemicals to somehow dissolve the shit on them before you wash them. That's really what you want in the corner of your kitchen - a mini sewage treatment plant. You can, if you're loaded, employ a nappy service. They will deliver a load of clean fresh terry cloth nappies to your home and take away the used ones for cleaning. Two things strike me about this. Firstly, while I haven't researched it I'm willing to bet it's pretty expensive and secondly, unless they collect the nappies every few hours you're still going to end up storing stinking nappies somewhere in your home.

Now you know what that distinctive new baby smell is: baby powder and faeces. I've just had a brainwave: that's going to be the name of my after shave range. What better way to attract women then to walk around smelling like the baby changing area in IKEA. I can see the TV ads now. A man walks into a bar smelling of baby powder and faeces. Every woman there starts to sniff the air and ovulate while every other man in the place runs out gagging. I'm going to be a millionaire.

Here's a fun fact. It's estimated that the average baby uses around five and a half thousand nappies before they are two and a half years old. All you environmentalists take note. That's a shitload of nappies (Was there ever a more apt collective noun?) If you pride yourself on being environmentally friendly you better go the terry nappy route or start nuking whales. Either way you won't be welcome at Greenpeace meetings anymore.

Help! I don't Want to Grow Up.

Who does? The one true joy of being a man is the fact that we never truly grow up. The good news is that kids help you to remain it touch with your inner brat. You get to revisit all those things you used to love but have forgotten all about. What about Lego? You used to love Lego. Many a happy hour was spent building castles, houses and fortresses and now you can do it all again. If you work in the construction industry you may not want to play with Lego. Who wants to stare at bricks all day and then come home and play with bricks? Play with yourself instead. In fact, to hell with Lego, let's go rent some porn.

Let's be completely honest here. You are immature beyond measure. You still think farts are hilarious, you only read crap books (ahem), you watch ridiculous action movies and if there's even a hint of a nipple around you'll stare at it like it was the Mona Lisa. Come to think of it, wouldn't the Mona Lisa be much better if her nipples were showing? Who gives a toss about her enigmatic smile or lack of eyebrows. If there was a wee nip slip over the top of her dress it would be the most famous picture in the world. Just like that one of the female tennis player scratching her arse. Let's start a campaign to get that one hanging in the Louvre. I've always thought that the Louvre sounds just like the loo so I always have a wee giggle when I hear that something was hanging in the Louvre. Same when I hear someone poncey saying that they could just spend hours in the Louvre. See, I told you men are immature.

So, do not worry your pretty little head about it. Major brain surgery and psychiatric intervention couldn't make you grow up. Constant nagging from Her couldn't make you grow up so what makes you think something that pees on you and laughs can do it. Simple answer is you'll never grow up. You'll be the wrinkliest guy on the seesaw in a few years.

Doula

A doula is someone, usually a woman, with no specific medical knowledge who is there to help Her during labour and post partum. It comes from a Greek word meaning female slave. I wish I had a few doulas. I don't recommend you say that though.

How Big a Life Change can I Expect?

Later we will talk about the joys of sleep deprivation, the lack of sex and the changes to the woman you love but I'm sorry to be the one to tell you this but there's a whole basket load of changes on top of all that. The actual arrival of the baby is really the beginning of the end for you. Your life as you knew it is over. There are things which you will miss terribly, Afternoon piss ups and general freedom to name but two. One friend of mine who was the first one in our circle to have kids told me around three months in that having a baby turns small things into huge chores. He used the example of returning a DVD to the rental store. Before baby it was a simple matter of jumping in the car, driving for five minutes, strolling into the DVD store and dropping it off. Hop back in the car and drive home. Total time elapsed: 10 minutes. With a baby however you have to dress the baby, put it in its car seat, put the baby in the car, get the changing bag, and drive the five minutes to the store. Take the baby out of the car, drop back the DVD, put the baby back in the car, drive home, take the baby out of the car, into the house and take off some of the layers of clothes on baby. Total time elapsed: 35 minutes.

Now, for the less mathematically able of you out there that means that one simple chore now takes over three times as long as it used to. Do you find that you have three times the amount of time you need each day? I thought not. So there's the first of it. Babies eat up more of your time than porn does. (You know how much time you spend looking at porn. Dirty bird).

There's also the huge financial element to consider. I went into money in detail in a separate section but suffice it to say that after your time and your energy levels money is the other thing the wee parasite...I mean, bundle of kitten fluff, drains away. So you have no time, no energy and no money. Is there anything that you gain from having a baby?

There is one thing you do get. I know this is going to sound hippyish or worse spiritual but one thing the baby will give you in return for everything you own, hope for and dream about is joy. I know that's not a word you say every day (unless you know someone named Joy obviously). Joy is a feeling I never had before I had kids. It's weird but it's the only word I can use to describe the feelings I get when I'm around my boys. Not all the time obviously. Not even one tenth of the time but God it's addictive. Sometimes, and you're never sure when, you just get this feeling which I can only describe as joy just from looking at your child. They will do something so unimaginably cute or they will say something amazing or even just look at you in a way which fills you up with the warmest, strongest feeling of happiness you've ever discovered.

Okay, I know I went a bit gooey there but hey, sue me. You'll do the same. Just take it from someone who's been there. Don't try to express these feelings to your friends or colleagues. They won't understand it and they will either take the piss mercilessly if they are your friends and if it's your co-workers they will probably not invite you to the next team building day. On second thought, tell your co-workers. Who wants to go running around in the woods shooting their colleagues with paintballs? On third thought. Don't tell your colleagues. It's more fun to go and shoot "Bubbly" Jackie from accounts or "Mad" Dave from marketing. They both deserve a bullet.

You'll experience this amazing feeling and the only one you can share it with is Her. That's okay though because she gets it and sometimes the greatest moments as parents is sitting together going all gooey over your kids. So, to put it simply, your life is going to be pretty much unrecognisable from the one you have now but you won't change back for anything

Top Five Jobs Pregnant Women Should Never Do

1. Roller Coaster Tester
2. Hostage Negotiator
3. Food Taster
4. Pole Dancer
5. Circumciser

Thoughts You Wish You Didn't Have

"I don't want to be a father!" Oh, the big one. This may have been unplanned or you may have agreed to try just to shut her up but secretly believed it would never happen. Now it has and you just don't want to go through with it. You see this as the end of your life. You look around at the hangdog look that you see on other fathers faces when they're struggling with kids and buggies and snot. You see the exhausted slightly spacey look on the faces of new dads who look like they would rather die than change another foul smelling nappy and give everything they own for eight hours of uninterrupted sleep. You've heard all the horror stories of colicky babies and genuine exhaustion (as opposed to got in from a party three hours before work exhaustion). You just don't want to face all that.

Well, good news and bad news. The bad news is that it's too late. Remember way back at the start when we laid down the ground rules? Remember number three? I made the assumption that you love Her so for that reason I know you aren't going to abandon Her and It so, as I say; basically you're screwed. Barring accident or injury you're going to be a father whether you like it or not. That's the bad news out of the way so before you try to paper cut your wrists here's the good news.

It's not even a quarter as hard or as awful as you imagine. The reason you've heard all the stories of screaming colicky babies and nightmare kids is because they make good stories. Oh, I'm not denying any of them but when was the last time you heard someone rattle on about how good their kids were as babies? Why do you think the news only reports the most awful stories? People don't pass on good news and stories but we relish bad ones. Why don't the police ever pull you over to tell you that you've been driving really well? The reason the dad you see with the buggy, screaming kids and snot look so depressed is because he's out with screaming kids. you don't see him when he's sitting in his garden while the kids run around or lying on the couch with his kids curled up to him watching a movie.

I remember being in Heathrow Airport in London around 15 years ago and watching this man walking with two kids, a Teletubby and the most exhaustedly morose look on his face and I remember thinking that I never want to have kids. When I learned that I was unexpectedly going to be a father for the first time that face returned and I will admit haunted my thoughts for a while. It's only now with the benefit of hindsight and experience that I realised of course the man looked morose and exhausted. Half the people in the airport looked like that. He had probably just stepped off a seven hour flight. Even without kids you look like crap after that and you certainly aren't feeling chirpy.

I'm not saying it's easy - far from it. There will be times when you'll curse my name for being so positive but it's certainly not the nightmare journey some make it out to be. Usually it's because they relish the horrified look on your face when you hear it. Remember that in this case you can't trust your mates. Think about it. If the shoe was on the other foot wouldn't you try to scar your mates with the most graphically horrible baby and birth stories you could find? Of course you would. You probably have and if you haven't believe me, the next one of your mates to become a father is going to be horrified by the stories you tell him. Like so many men before you, you will embellish and downright lie just to wind them up. Trust me, it's much more fun giving than receiving in this case (and in anal sex I'm guessing). So don't worry about not wanting to be a father. No one in their right mind wants to be a father. What sane young man wants to give up freedom and cold hard cash? No one. However, sane young men have no idea what the reality of being a father is. No sane father would ever want to trade places with a sane young man. Well, maybe for a few weeks a year, and the odd weekend and while we're at it, can I have a bigger dick too?

Montgomery's Tubercules

Raised lumps which appear on the aureolas of pregnant women. Discovered by Montgomery who described them as "A constellation of nipples scattered over a milky way." That guy was either a legend or mad as fuck - either way he made a living from looking at boobies so he wasn't stupid.

Just whose boobs are they anyway?

We talked earlier about that most glorious of days, the arrival of the Booby Fairy. As I said, the booby Fairy arrives in the night and gives you a wonderful gift: the gift of new, bigger boobs. This is a wonderful gift but also a double edged sword. While you are standing there admiring these new wonders She may well be feeling nauseous thanks to morning sickness and the boobs themselves may be sore. She may not want you touching them. She may not even want you looking at them. These changes have to be freaking her out.

Imagine if you woke up in the morning to find your willie considerably bigger. Okay, bad example, you'd be delighted. Okay imagine it was bigger and too sore to touch. Oh cruel irony. Imagine it was bigger, too sore to touch and She kept pawing at it every time you stood at the sink washing up. You know what? Screw it. I'd still be delighted and so would you if you're honest. There are some excellent painkillers on the market. The penis is an odd thing anyway. You never know just how big it's going to get on any given outing (I just realised that last sentence made me sound like a flasher). I mean that depending on mood, stimulation, temperature and moon alignment your manhood can vary in length, girth and rigidity. We're always pleasantly surprised when we get an unexpectedly huge one but we've derived pleasure from it in nearly all stages so quite frankly we're happy just to own one. A woman's body image is much more fragile so give her time to get used to the changes. You will be rewarded eventually with a few goes on the new playtime activity centre that is her body.

Serious time: you may be freaked out by all the changes in her body. I mentioned earlier about how I was freaked out when I learned that my wife's nipples were going to darken. I know it seems trite but until that moment I hadn't considered that the changes to her body could affect me. I knew she was going to get bigger and that she was going to put on weight but I somehow imagined that after birth everything would go back to normal. For the most part it does but there are still some permanent changes.

Let's look at the worst case scenarios and deal with your worst fears. Number one on most guys list is that she will get very loose down there after giving birth. Of course she will. It's going to stretch wide enough to accommodate a baby's head and no matter how delusional you are, even you have to admit that you don't stack up to that.

She may experience some tearing which is exactly as it sounds. Sometimes the doctor will elect to give her an episiotomy which is where they make a surgical cut. The reason why they do this is to avoid tearing. A neat surgical cut is a lot easier to stitch up and heal than a tear. There are different levels of tearing. I won't go into details here. You don't need to know the eye watering specifics. Suffice it to say that even without any tearing or cutting after the birth she'll probably look like the sleeve of a woollen jumper straight out of the washing machine. The good news is that with proper care and exercises everything should go back to normal and your tiny member will feel like a porn stars weapon once more.

Notice I mentioned proper care and exercise. I mean pelvic floor exercises also known as "Kegels", named after the guy who devised them. Kegels should be done by her in the weeks leading up to birth as it helps prepare the pelvic floor. They should then be done after the birth to get the vagina back to its old grippy ways. You can do Kegels too. They help to give you stronger thicker erections.

Wait a minute, what? Yep, Kegels give you bigger, thicker, stronger erections. They work by strengthening the pubococcygeal muscles. A simple exercise for you is this. You know when you are taking a pee in a neighbour's garden on the way home from the pub and you hear their back door open? We've all been there. When you desperately clamp your urethra shut it's the pubococcygeal muscles that do that. Try tensing them now. There you go. Now, do that thirty times twice a day and wait for your new, stronger erections to appear. How about that. I just delivered on all the false promises your spam filter shelters you from. I'm deadly serious, do those exercises and your manhood will improve. You're welcome. Now that you're doing them, its time to work on her.

Kegels are incredibly effective but the trick is getting her to do them diplomatically. I don't mean carrying a tray of gold wrapped chocolate testicles through the ambassador's reception. I mean that she will be exhausted and sore and the last thing she's thinking about is sex or exercise. No woman wants to lose tightness and if you asked her about it when she was relaxed, with a glass of wine or two de-stressing her she would freely admit that. Walking up to her and saying "I hope you're doing your fanny exercises. I don't want to fall in" is never going to lead to a grateful kiss on the cheek for your gentle reminder. The best thing you can do here is talk to her and be open and honest. I know that you recognise those words as English but have never seen them in that particular order before. Yes, it's possible to be open and honest with your feelings. If it makes it any easier pretend to yourself that you're lying or relaying a movie plot you saw once.

Whatever trick you use, choose your time wisely. Pick a time when the baby is asleep and she appears relaxed. Tell her how great you think she's doing as a mother and rub her feet or something. Gently nudge the conversation towards your relationship with each other and mention that you're afraid to hurt her the next time you have sex. She will reassure you that you won't and that in a few weeks everything will be back to normal. Now for the finesse: ask her if she is worried about anything sexually. Is she worried about getting hurt or leaking boobs or loss of tightness? See what I did there? You're now talking about her lady garden and you don't look like an insensitive asshole. The conversation should flow towards pelvic floor exercises and Kegels (same thing really). Tell her that you've been doing this because you know how important a healthy sex life is for a couple. The fact that you are doing exercises too shows solidarity with her that she'll really appreciate. It doesn't matter that you only want to look good in Speedos on your next holiday. She'll never know that. You have now planted a seed so get the fuck out of the garden before you say something stupid which leads to a month of sleeping on the sofa. In all seriousness, gently encourage her to exercise and remind both of you that you are sexual beings and you will have sex again.

Another fear that most men have is that she'll never lose the weight she put on during pregnancy. Well, that's a possibility. At the very least, give her time. She will be exhausted and you know why. Let her keep eating like a rescued castaway for as long as it takes. She will be aware of her body much more than you are but as we all know its hard enough motivating yourself to exercise even when you're not clinically exhausted. Give her time to get used to the baby and recover from pregnancy and labour and then it's time for another one of those open and honest chats. I know, I never said this was going to be easy. Same scenario as before: make sure she's rested and relaxed and then best of luck.

Listen, I know a fair bit about pregnancy and childbirth but if I knew how to delicately encourage a woman to lose weight without getting torn limb from limb I'd be God, I would be a multi-billionaire and have the love and respect of every man on the planet. Tell her you love her no matter what. Whatever you say next is up to you. You have my prayers and the hopes and fears of all mankind resting on you. Good luck.

You may worry that her boobs will go all droopy like some tribeswoman on a National Geographic special and that's normal too. The truth is she may not be as firm as before but dude, they're boobs. You love boobs. I defy you to remember what her boobs looked like before pregnancy. You will love these boobs as much as her old ones because you're a man and grateful for any boob contact at all. Honestly, the change won't be as dramatic or noticeable as you imagine. Now milk coming out of them: that's a whole different kettle of fish. Whether a woman breastfeeds or not her body will, for a time be producing breast milk. You may be freaked out, turned on or grossed out completely by the idea of lactation. Whichever dairy you fall into is okay. I shouldn't tell you this but if you squeeze her boobs just right you can get them to squirt milk like a water pistol. How's that for a way of chasing the neighbourhood kids out of your garden?

Stevie's month by month guide to the creature inside her: 3rd month

Your baby is growing much faster now. Its length is around seven centimetres and is around the size of an apple. It looks just like a foetus and you can even tell its sex if you squint. Freaky fact: it's producing urine now and peeing inside your missus. Gross.

Once while having sex I forgot myself and squeezed her boob. She was on top and I made the perfect shot as milk shot out of her and got me right in the eye. If you saw it in a movie you'd say it was too far fetched. Mind you, what sort of movies do you watch dude. Seriously, not cool. The point is, I got a shot in the face (some would call that poetic justice) and it was gross but guess what? I finished off just fine. Sure I didn't like it but it was breast milk. I'm a man; it would have had to have been acid to put me off. What I'm saying is if you're freaked out or grossed out by breast milk it's possible to avoid it but if the worst should happen you are a man and its only milk so either wipe your face on the duvet and keep going or chuck in some Coco Pops and have fun. Now that I've alleviated all your fears lets move on.

Okay, I'll sum up for you. You both probably plan on growing old together. Neither you nor her imagined that your bodies would remain the same did you? While you're sitting there lamenting the droop of her boobs or the width of her arse do you think you're not changing too? A lot of men put on a load of weight during pregnancy and for the first few months. You're exhausted too and you'll comfort eat. Believe me, the physical changes to you both are really the smallest of the life changes that come with having children so accept the physical changes for now. Some will soon be a distant memory while others will become permanent. Either way, you will find her sexy, she will turn you on and sex, when you can have it, will be better than ever.

Will She ever stop puking?

Morning sickness: something those of you with an over dependence on alcohol will be all too familiar with. The big difference is that She doesn't get the joy of getting hammered the night before. It's one of those pregnancy symptoms which are so accepted that we forget just how horrible it is. Imagine having a hangover for months. Months! Spending each day feeling at best nauseous and at worst blowing chunks every time someone farts on TV (something which there needs to be more of on TV in my opinion. Seriously, when did you last hear a good fart on TV? The world as I knew it has moved on. Sigh.) It really does make her miserable and just because loads of pregnant women experience it doesn't make it any less awful.

What one piece of advice would you give to a man on how to handle his pregnant partner?

Her hormones are flying around her like never before so be on good behaviour. Keep a record of everything you do or say during the pregnancy because she'll constantly remind you of all the things you didn't do to help her for years afterwards. Women get a surge of hormones for the second trimester to help them through the nesting period and they get loads done but she'll look back and think "I was PREGNANT and I painted all the bedrooms and drove around looking for prams and he just sat there, the bastard".

Patrick, Comedian and Actor

The simple facts of morning sickness are these: Morning sickness is commonly the first sign of pregnancy. More than half of all women suffer from it. It usually manifests itself around the sixth week of pregnancy, but can occur as early as four, and flushes away after the twelfth, although sometimes as far as the fourteenth (some unlucky women experience it for almost the entire pregnancy. For the love of God don't tell her that.). Despite the name, morning sickness can strike at any time of the day although it is common for Her to feel nauseated in the morning and have the symptoms ease as the day progresses. Not all women puke however, some just feel nauseous. As with so much to do with pregnancy, the jury is still out as to the actual cause of morning sickness. Theories about increased oestrogen levels dance freely with laying the blame at the pregnant one's increased sensitivity to odours. (That includes your fetid morning breath by the way).

One theory which is gaining increasing credence is that morning sickness is a defence mechanism to protect the foetus. Here's the layman's (i.e. us) version; morning sickness is an evolved trait which helps protect the foetus from toxins which the mother may ingest. These toxins are present in a number of foods and are completely harmless to us but which the foetus hasn't built up an immunity to yet. The woman eats something which may harm the foetus and the body rejects it. One fact which supports this theory is that the foetus' immunity to toxins is established by the third month which is commonly when morning sickness stops. Pretty cool huh? So the next time She's ass in the air/head down the bowl making noises like an asthmatic warthog you can tell her about the great job she's doing protecting the baby. Semper fi love, semper fi.

So Stevie, fount of all knowledge, what can I do? Well, as usual try not to take the piss too much. She's really suffering here and could do with your support. Encourage her to eat six small meals instead of three large ones. Some women swear by eating crackers in the morning. The smell of lemons can help so encourage her to keep on with the washing up. Chop up some fresh root ginger and put it in boiling water. Let it cool a bit and have her sip it until the nausea passes. Ginger is great for any type of tummy upset. Try it yourself. Hiring a stripper named Ginger may not be as effective but hey, you'll try anything to help Her feel better. On a positive note: one recent study has shown that women who don't suffer from morning sickness have an increased risk of miscarriage and birth defects. This backs up the toxin defence theory. If She isn't suffering from morning sickness don't go running off thinking that something will go wrong. I only say this so that if She is being sick you can drop that nugget on her which might make Her feel a tiny bit better. I don't have to tell you not to say a word to Her if She's not sick.

Things to do with Preggo No. 1

Try doing a photo a day record of her pregnancy. Then print them out and use them like a flicker book. Watch the woman you love balloon or run it backwards and watch her go back to normal. Her boobs shrink though. For God's sake though get Her to smile for the photos. I know of one woman who didn't. It put me in mind of a death row prisoner who gets to eat a last meal for every meal.

CHAPTER 2

THE SEVEN HORMONAL DWARVES

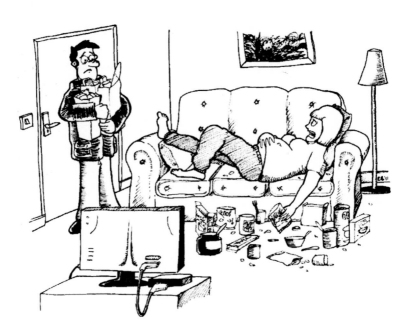

"You'd better have managed to get me a woolly mammoth burger"

She Can't be Hungry Again!

It's twelve thirty at night and you are frantically miming to an overnight petrol station attendant. You are trying to ask for beef jerky without being too obscene in your gestures and he's looking at you with that peculiar disdain that only someone working the graveyard shift can muster. They've seen it all: the drunks, the stoners and of course the most desperate of all…the guys trying to satisfy the near impossible cravings of a pregnant woman.

It's estimated that around sixty eight percent of pregnant women suffer from pregnancy cravings. Well, I say suffer. Some women suffer, the women who crave non food items or revolting food combinations suffer. Some women however crave chocolate or cheeseburgers. Well guess what? So do I. The difference is that if I started scarfing down treats at three AM people would start calling me a pig and no one would want to carry my incredibly oversized coffin when I eventually died of a heart attack while desperately trying to open a tube of Pringles. Don't get me wrong, pregnancy cravings are real and sixty eight percent of women suffer from them. I'm just saying that some of that percentage are incredibly lucky that they happen to crave only their favourite foods. How very, very convenient. Just saying.

For the majority however, the cravings are as real as the chain smokers desperate first gasp of nicotine in the morning. There is no one universally accepted theory as to why women experience cravings. Some believe that it's down to a deficiency in certain nutrients and that specific foods answer different needs. Others believe that it is in response to the trauma of morning sickness as cravings usually manifest themselves when sickness clears. I believe that women like to make men offer constant reassurance while pregnant. What better way is there of saying I love you than returning home at midnight with a jar of pimento stuffed olives and a family sized box of After Eights. The primitive cave woman part of her brain is now secure in the knowledge that her hunter gatherer mate will provide for the baby. Just be glad that mammoths and sabre toothed tigers are extinct or she'd want a couple of pizzas made out of them too.

When most people think of pregnancy cravings they think of the infamous pickles and ice cream combination. I have to say that although I've never tried that it sounds kind of great. The saltiness of the pickles followed by the sweet cold of the ice cream ...Just a sec, I'll be back in a minute.

I'm back. You may not believe this but while I was writing that last piece I remembered that we had a jar of pickles in the fridge. Off I went and lo and behold we had both a jar of pickles and a large tub of vanilla ice cream. Let me say, I take back all I said. Pickles and ice cream are a horrible combination. Why anyone would voluntarily inflict that particular taste combination on themselves is beyond me. I read a book once where a woman was carrying a demons baby and it used to make her go out at night and eat live frogs. She'd wake in the morning with no recollection of the previous night but with incredibly dirty feet. Not that I'm saying your baby is a demon but perhaps check it's scalp for sixes after It's born.

Pregnancy cravings are 100% genuine and it's your job to satisfy them. Make sure the car is gassed up, that you have all the local fast food joints programmed into the SatNav and most importantly, that you have the personal home numbers of the owners and staff so that you can get them to open up at four a.m. in case they're needed. The cravings are real and believe me its better to have a post midnight dash to the 24 hour supermarket than a visit from Angry and Furious.

The other side of the cravings coin is called Pica which is the Latin word for Magpie (a bird notorious for eating anything) and is the unfortunate condition where the woman craves non food items such as dirt, matches or laundry detergent. There are different types of Pica and some are more dangerous than others. Pagophagia for example is the relatively harmless craving for ice while Amylophagia is the craving for starch and paste. This is one of the more dangerous cravings due to the risk of blockage or the toxicity of the items themselves. There is a fear that women can be reluctant to tell their doctor if they are experiencing Pica due to embarrassment. Geophagia for example is the consumption of earth and clay. Some believe that it can combat the nausea of morning sickness.

Weirdly, this form of craving is most common in Central Africa and the Southern United States and may have some cultural connotations. This is another area where being aware of what

She is going through could really help protect her. Any changes in bowel movements or distention of the abdomen other than normal pregnancy changes should be reported to her doctor. While it is rare it's not uncommon for this condition to lead to serious injury or even death.

So, whatever She craves is your Holy Grail. If you are lucky She might crave grass and that will mean a perfect lawn for you all summer long. Whatever the craving, there is no greater sound than the happy munching of a newly satiated pregnant woman with a lap full of goodies and TV full of rubbish. So, get out there brave knight. Do whatever you must to return with her bounty (it might actually be a Bounty) and fair maid shall grant thee the greatest boon of all. A bit of peace. (At least until She's hungry again).

Stevie's month by month guide to the creature inside her: 4th month

Your baby is growing faster and faster. It's around four inches long and even has fingerprints, so no crime sprees with the foetus okay? Freaky fact, it's covered in hair now. It'll fall out well before the birth but still; it resembles a monkey more than ever now. Resist the urge to stick a banana up there.

I can't stand OPC (Other Peoples Children) how will I tolerate my own?

There is a great old expression that goes, "Kids are like farts. You can barely stand your own." I love that. Not least, because it's true. Maybe it's a male thing but I can spot an ugly baby from 500 metres while my wife thinks every kid on the planet is adorable. I have never raised a hand to my kids but I don't think I would have a problem with beating the snot out of anyone else's. Don't worry if you can't stand kids. That's normal. Kids are a pain in the ass pretty much all the time. Even yours will be. The difference is you love yours so you can tolerate it. I personally find my kids friends annoying at best.

By the way, you and Her are the only ones who will appreciate the wondrous actions, looks or sounds of your baby. Don't make the rookie mistake of thinking everyone thinks your baby is as adorable as you do. Have you ever looked at someone else's kids and thought "Woof. That is one ugly baby." Do you think that they see an ugly kid when they look at him? Of course not, they think that horror movie extra that is their kid is a shoo-in to win the local bonny baby competition. You know he'd have a better chance of entering a Halloween costume competition. I'm lucky in that my kids actually are stunningly good looking but you'd be amazed at the amount of delusional people there are out there.

Another thing you'll notice very quickly is that no matter what your baby does, whoever you say it to, their baby will have done the same thing earlier and better than your baby. There is only one defence here. Lie. Lie like you've come home from the pub with a phone number written in lipstick on your ass, (Actually happened to a guy I know. We did it to him while he was passed out. I wonder if he and the wife ever got back together?) It's okay to lie to other parents about your child's development because they sure as hell are lying to you. If parents were to be believed every kid on the planet was walking five minutes after leaving the womb and spoke four languages by the time they were weaned onto solid food. They even prepared the food. Hell, they went out and bought the ingredients and paid for them with the money they earned from working for NASA.

To lie effectively, wait until the other parents, or The Enemy as they shall henceforth be known, offers some boast about their little prodigy and just one up them. If they say their baby walked at nine months tell them yours actually walked out of the womb and asked for someone to cut the cord so it could go get a shower. If they say their baby was talking at twelve months tell them that your baby actually phoned from the womb to tell them he was on his way out. Keep your lies believable, that's the trick.

What the Hell is She Wearing?

Q: What do spacesuits and pregnancy jeans have in common?
A: They both have to be able to withstand extreme pressure and they sure as hell aren't flattering.

Let's' get one thing straight before we go on. There is absolutely nothing sexy about maternity clothes. She can look pretty, classy, professional, even athletic. (Okay, not athletic in the Olympic sense, more Mount Olympus, but you get the idea). The one thing they are not is sexy. Lets go through the changes that are about to occur in her wardrobe but believe me there will be some things in there soon that would make finding Narnia back there seem normal.

First there are pregnancy jeans. These are a marvel of design. I'm guessing that polar expedition suits have had less thought and testing put into them than your average balloon arsed, stretchy panelled denim duvet that is the pregnancy jean. I will admit that there is an element of jealousy creeping in here because despite how much I rail against them I can't help but stare and think about just how incredibly comfy they look. No belt, no braces, no tight button and no zip just a huge expanse of stretchy cloth that moulds itself to your belly and simply defies gravity. How great would it be to wander around all day proudly displaying your beer gut instead of holding your breath every time a woman is within fifty feet? How great to have trousers that never remind you of how much weight you're putting on because they stretch to fit even the most portly of bodies? Finally getting the chance to say; screw you to fashion and a big howdy-do to middle age. It would be heaven on Earth. However, if we did wear pregnancy jeans do you think anyone would ever have sex with us again? Of course not. Comfy things are not sexy and pregnant women want, and deserve, to wear comfy clothes throughout pregnancy.

So pregnancy jeans and dungarees are about as appealing as a thick lustrous moustache is on either sex. If She wore a pair of pregnancy dungarees, a straw hat and carried a bag you could easily imagine her picking up rubbish on Wimbledon Common. ("Underground, over ground" etc. Look it up)

What about those pretty maternity dresses you see happy pregnant models wearing in magazines? I hear you cry. Surely they exist. Only in the fetid dreams of the advertisers my friend. I've always suspected that those pregnant models aren't pregnant at all. They are just wearing fake bumps or something. There's no way on Earth that you can keep a pregnant woman smiling for the entire length of a photo shoot. It's hard enough to keep monumentally stoned models feeling chirpy let alone a tired, hormonal woman who feels about as sexy as a chest freezer. She will never look like the professionals in those outfits but she'll try and that is the sweetest thing of all. But then, what if the roles were reversed? Imagine you were trying to fit into your old PE kit from secondary school. How well do you think it would fit today? Are you pregnant? No? Well then, give her a break. This is another one of those side effects she never asked for yet has to live with throughout this pregnancy. Tell her ten times a day how beautiful She looks. She will scoff and tell you you're blind but inside she'll feel a lot better about herself.

Feeling frisky? There is a huge market in pregnancy lingerie. There is also a huge market in pregnancy knickers. To us these are the same but to her however there is a world of difference. A simple rule of thumb is this: pregnancy lingerie pays some lip service to looking sexy while pregnancy knickers just don't bother. To be honest, if pregnancy knickers tried to look sexy they would fail so dismally that it would make the captain of the Titanic's decision to let Cross-Eyed Joe take first lookout seem intelligent. Pregnancy knickers are designed to control, conceal, absorb and effectively cover a pregnant woman's shame. Pregnancy lingerie's remit is somewhat smaller. It's there to make her feel, not look, sexy. Your job is to tell her that she looks hotter than a fat guy on a sun holiday chasing an ice cream truck while eating a bowl of extra hot chilli (I've seen something remarkably similar).

Can you believe that they now make thongs in sizes up to and including size thirty two? I'm sorry but if you are wearing a size thirty two thong then you look like you're wearing normal knickers, just that you've absorbed them. I've always felt that tracksuits should only be in athlete's sizes just to stop the morbidly obese from getting bigger and that lingerie should have a size limit or come with a warning over a certain size.

Imagine finding the following written on a maternity bra; Objects contained within may be larger than they appear or on a pair of maternity knickers; Contents under extreme pressure and liable to emit gas. What a wonderful world this could be.

Pregnancy bras are truly a wonder of the modern age. They literally could support the world if gravity ever failed us. They can withstand forces equivalent to The Big Bang (Not the conception. Show off.) They are second only to the nursing bra in ingenuity. The nursing bra does everything the pregnancy bra does while being able to cope with any amount of leaking and with access panels on the front to allow quick and easy access to the boobies for baby. I'm sure you're asking yourself the same question as I am. If this technology exists, why don't all bras allow for such free and unfettered access? Why should babies have all the fun? It's probably because God hates us. He never got over the whole Garden of Eden/ Stop nicking my fruit debacle and so makes us work for every glimpse or feel of boob for our entire lives. It's original sin, pure and simple.

As I said earlier, pregnancy clothes can be many things but sexy isn't one of them. Never, ever tell her that. I hope you've learned by now just how fragile and dangerous a pregnant woman is. Any hint that you find her clothing amusing or off-putting will shatter her already strained ego to the point that all the worst of the dwarves (remember them?) will come out to see what all the fuss is about. Sure, comparing her to one of the Wombles is hilarious at the time but as far as I know Great Uncle Bulgaria never tore the testicles off some unsuspecting man on Wimbledon Common. Don't let you be the first.

Genuine Names of Pregnancy Lingerie Collections

1. Wild Composure: Never before has pregnancy been described so eloquently.
2. Blissful Disorder: Another good pregnancy analogy.
3. Quiet Storm: Okay, now they're taking the piss.
4. Ruffle My Feathers: No way. I know what pregnant women are like when you ruffle their feathers. Happy chicks can become Angry Birds in a second.
5. Slip into Seduction: Pregnant women don't slip into anything. Plonk gratefully into Seduction would be more apt.

Why Does She Seem a bit Dumber than Normal?

Some aspects of pregnancy are harder to deal with than others. Body changes, insomnia and countless embarrassing ailments all take their toll on Her and you. There is one condition however which is fun at least and downright handy at times. I am talking about Pregnancy Brain. This is a genuine, documented condition caused as usual by hormones which leads to forgetfulness and a general dullness of the brain. During the third trimester She actually has a lower volume of brain cells than normal and this leads to many "senior moments". The good news is that a few months after the birth She will be as sharp as ever. However while She's a bit ditzy, this is your time for some mischief.

You amateurs can use this time to play tricks on Her such as hiding Her car keys or putting one of Her shoes on the roof. The sneakier among you can use this forgetfulness to your advantage. "But you said I could go to the game with the lads" or "You said that if I did the dishes we could have a threesome with your best mate." The only limit here is your imagination.

In all seriousness your job here is to help her have a sense of humour about it and to make sure you don't entrust her with the nuclear activation codes. Encourage Her to write important things down in huge letters and to display them prominently. Get Her to use her phone as an organiser which can really help provided She can find the phone when She needs it. This is far from the end of the world but it's another element to be aware of. You never know, you just might get that threesome after all. It's just a pity She probably won't remember it. Mind you, as long as you do who cares?

Top Five Most Popular Female Porn Star Names

    6.   Jenna
    7.   Rachael
    8.   Angelina
    9.   Holly
  10. Savannah

Are there any benefits to this pregnancy lark?

Apart from creating new life you mean? Is that not enough for you? Honestly, sometimes I don't know why I bother.

Yes, there are benefits. You just have to recognise them and seize every opportunity. Let's look at a few of the simpler ones: First of all you won't have to drive home from any nights out for a while. You can magnanimously offer to drive to the party, get hammered and get driven home by the world's most resentful chauffeur. A word of warning however: remember just how much she hates to see you enjoying yourself when She isn't. You're dancing the Macarena on a friend's lawn while She's sitting in the car quietly seething and preparing for a long drive with a captive audience for Her nagging. She will be sick of being the sober one so the sight of you with a boozy grin plastered all over your face is bound to get on her nerves.

You can make the trip home much more fun for both of you by following these simple rules.
- Take this opportunity to offer Her pointers on Her driving. You are ideally placed to examine and evaluate Her driving technique so feel free. She'll really appreciate the benefit of your superior driving knowledge.
- Make sure to use this time to make gestures towards other, less able drivers. She'll be too busy trying to put into practice all the handy advice you've given Her and She'll appreciate you dealing with other road users on Her behalf.
- Make sure to change the radio station at least once or twice per minute to ensure that She's bang up to date with all the latest tunes.
- Finally, there may be times when She forgets to perform some simple signal such as indicating or dimming Her lights for oncoming motorists. This is probably due to pregnancy brain and obviously, Her gender. She'll really appreciate you reaching over and performing these tasks for Her. Nothing says I'm here for you, more than reaching across Her to the indicator stalk and sparing Her some embarrassment.

Now, if you're dumb enough to believe the above list then please never help your child with their homework. Nothing looks worse than an enthusiastic daddy colouring in his child's maths homework. While we're at it, let's leave any major decisions regarding your child's future to Her shall we? It's probably for the best. The more astute of you will have noticed that performing any of the actions on the above list will lead to you walking home at best and crawling home at worst. If you play this right, with breastfeeding etc. you should be able to get at least a year of free limo service. All you have to do is bite your tongue whenever She does something you wouldn't do while driving: like keeping to the speed limit or something crazy like that.

Another benefit to this whole baby making lark is the increased privacy it affords. To put it simply, pregnant women are a lot like hurricanes in that they've never managed to sneak up on anyone. Once She has settled down into bed for the night you can pretty much do whatever you like. If She wants to get up She gives more advance warning than a glacier attack. From the sounds of a bed creaking under severe strain to the gentle shuffle of her swollen, slipper clad feet to the inevitable stop for a pee before She even reaches the top of the stairs. All this ensures that you have more than enough time to remove all traces of whatever nefarious scheme you're involved in.

More than enough time to clear your browsing history, remove the incriminating DVD from the player. Hell, you could set up a meth lab in your living room and you'd have time to dismantle it and clear out all your customers before she was halfway down the stairs. So make hay, or meth, (Okay, don't make meth) while the sun shines and be glad of this "Me" time.

Things to do with Preggo No. 2

Get her to lie on her stomach and have local teens use her as a skateboard/BMX ramp. Alternatively see how many break-dance spins She can do on the bump. Get the local teens round for a dance off. It'll give you a chance to sell all that meth you made

One final benefit to Her being pregnant is quite a gooey one (Not that sort of gooey, Sicko. Gooey in a cute sense). Because of the extra attention you're focusing on Her at this time you get a chance to spend a greater amount of quality time together. You may have been the sort of couple who went out every weekend and once or twice during the week. This will obviously ease off, especially as the pregnancy draws towards the end. Because of this you naturally will be spending more time together and as you will be focusing on Her needs a lot it'll bring you both closer. Curling up with Her on the couch with a good movie and enough food to feed an army is great. Sitting with your hand on Her bump waiting for the baby to kick is even more so. Giving Her a foot rub is a pain in the arse (It's not all sunshine and flowers). So, to put it simply, the greatest benefit to pregnancy is that you get to spend more time with someone you love. Enjoy these moments together because pretty soon there will be at least three of you fighting for space on the couch but remember your natural role as guardian of the remote control. As constant as the sun rising in the east or the dishonesty of politicians, that will never change.

CHAPTER 3

MOTHER NATURE AND THE GRAPES OF ASS

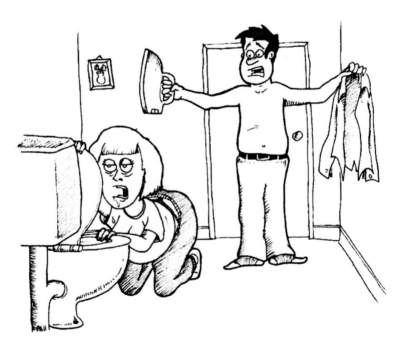

"Where did you tell me to shove these again?"

Eleven Common Ailments During Pregnancy

She is going to be prone to a number of embarrassing, annoying and sometimes painful afflictions throughout pregnancy and while you can obviously have a quiet, or not so quiet, giggle at the more embarrassing ones you can also do a fair bit to help. Below is a list of the top eleven most common ailments She may experience and what if anything you can do to help. I've alphabetised them to keep the OCD crowd happy.

1. Backache

Pregnant women are prone to backache not least because of the bowling ball they're carrying around. Sometime around the second trimester a hormone (Remember them?) called Relaxin, which is probably the coolest name for a hormone ever, is produced which helps the ligaments around the back and pelvis relax in preparation for childbirth. This can lead to quite severe backache and something like turning over in bed can be especially painful (so no Kama Sutra positions for a while).

How you can help:
You can help by giving her non-sexual massages (yes, they exist) and encouraging her to exercise. A cake on the end of a stick can help motivate her during this time. She should also avoid lifting anything heavy so it's best that you hold your own penis for now. (High five. Who's with me?)

2. Constipation

Funny, funny stuff constipation. Unless you're the one suffering from it of course. Thanks to our good old friend Progesterone (pity it's not a hormone called keepitin or bungabum). This is just one more side benefit of this particular hormone. Another cause can be an over abundance of iron. Iron is one of those minerals that a pregnant woman can become deficient in and often She will be given an iron supplement. Ironically (*iron*ically, get it? Sod you then) this can lead to constipation. Try encouraging her to have a big steak a couple of time a week. This is one of those times where you should lead by example. Obviously as an affliction it's painful and embarrassing but if left untreated can cause major problems. Not least of which is you legitimately telling Her that She's full of shit during an argument. Imagine the bloodshed.

How you can help:
Firstly, encourage her to drink loads of water and to eat more fruit and fibre. She can also try Senna which is all natural and completely safe for her to take. If She is going to use an over the counter laxative from a pharmacist, make sure of two things. Firstly make sure to tell the pharmacist that it's for a pregnant woman and secondly make sure that you go and buy it for her. She has enough embarrassment to deal with during pregnancy without having to describe her bowel movements to some teenager on work experience.

3.   Cramps

Cramps. These are what you'd call a bastard. She may experience incredibly painful leg cramps. They usually occur at night and begin after the 20th week of pregnancy. They are believed to be caused by a deficiency in Calcium and Magnesium which the baby is absorbing like a hungry vampire.

How you can help:
While you're getting her laxatives from the pharmacist pick Her up a supplement which obviously is safe for a pregnant woman to take. Make sure that She drinks plenty of water and gets some exercise during the day. Also encourage Her to wear flat shoes so unfortunately, no stripper heels until after the baby is born. Okay, maybe for the birth. Why not get her to throw on some nipple tassels while She's at it.

4.   Fluid Retention

This does not mean She's going to confiscate your beer or that She could now drink you under the table. Pregnant women swell up (not just her ass. Grow up!) It is common for a pregnant woman's ankles and feet to swell up late in the afternoon especially during hot weather. When this is more pronounced it can lead to Oedema. Oedema means swelling and can be caused by very hot weather or standing in one place for long periods. In itself it's not considered dangerous but it is an indicator of potential pre-eclampsia, a much more serious condition which requires hospitalisation. If Oedema is severe a trip to Her doctor to check Her blood pressure is recommended.

How you can help:
As usual your vigilance counts. If you notice Her hands, feet, ankles face and neck swelling up. Firstly make sure that you are not in Willy Wonka's Chocolate Factory and She has eaten some experimental sweetie. If not then check for pitting. This is where you apply pressure with a finger to an area of swelling (Honestly, I am giggling away as I write this at the double meanings here) for 20-30 seconds. After you remove your finger there should be an obvious dent which you can both see and feel. This is a good indicator of Oedema and off to the doctor you go. Make sure She gets plenty of rest in the evenings, preferably with Her feet raised. Resist the urge to watch documentaries about Bigfoot and try not to make toad noises whenever She looks down.

5.   Haemorrhoids

Back to the funnies. Okay, let's get this out of the way. Haemorrhoids are funny as hell. I can think of no fewer than five million pain in the arse/these grapes taste funny jokes as soon as I hear the word. So let's get all the puerile ass gags out of our systems now because if you are the one suffering from them they really aren't funny at all. Haemorrhoids are basically varicose veins of the anus (Damn it. Even that sentence is funny.) Our old buddy Progesterone relaxes the blood vessels and as the uterus grows it applies pressure and then the vineyard can expect a good harvest (Last one. I promise). They can also be caused by straining from constipation so go back up to number two (if you'll pardon the pun) and bone up.
Some of the symptoms of haemorrhoids are obvious. pain or severe itching around the anus. There can also be a small amount of fresh blood, this is usually noticed as spotting on toilet tissue when having a bowel movement. There may also be some form of mucus discharge (could pregnancy be any sexier?)

How you can help:
While painful and embarrassing, haemorrhoids are relatively easy to treat. Natural remedies such as witch-hazel tincture and tissue salts are available from your pharmacy but most

haemorrhoid treatments are safe for use by pregnant women but as usual check with the pharmacist. You main job here is to go buy whatever treatment She decides to use. This is to spare Her blushes. Make a game of it. Walk like an old time cowboy and wince as you approach the counter. You could also get her a haemorrhoid doughnut. This is not the world's most unappetising dessert. This is an inflatable ring for her to sit on which allows her dangleberries to sway gently in the breeze. (I'm a poet). Once again keep your eyes peeled. If She notices that the blood in her bowel movements is dark in colour or if the symptoms persist for longer than two weeks get her to consult with her doctor.

6. Heartburn

Heartburn, or acid reflux as it is also known, is caused by, you guessed it, Progesterone. It relaxes the valve at the entrance to the stomach so it's easier for stomach acid to flow into the oesophagus causing that distinctive burning pain. She usually experiences it when she's coughing, straining or commonly while she's lying down. Also the baby can sometimes press on Her stomach which causes a mini stomach acid tsunami. Whatever the cause it's quite painful and because it's common when She is lying down it can really affect Her sleep.

How you can help:
Encourage her to eat smaller meals but more frequently as large meals exacerbate the condition. Also try to discourage her from eating spicy foods or foods high in fat. (Good luck with that). A glass of milk or antacids can alleviate the symptoms. As usual, check with Her doctor. Propping her up in bed with loads of pillows can help too so give up your pillow and win back some of the brownie points you lost when laughing at her haemorrhoids.

7. Insomnia

One of the more horribly cruel ironies of pregnancy is that when its over you can't sleep because you're looking after a newborn baby yet during pregnancy you may not get much rest either. It's like asking a marathon runner to jog to the Olympics on the day of the big race. Sleeplessness can be caused by a number of factors during pregnancy. We've discussed heartburn and leg cramps but there is also the wee creature itself. Not your personal wee creature and its insane demands. No, the wee creature growing inside her has his own clock and likes company so he may start doing the can-can at three am and demand She stays awake to enjoy the show.

How you can help:
Any natural sleep remedy you can think of for a start. Chamomile tea, massage, soft lighting, whale noises. Try everything you can think of because She can't take sleeping pills. The good news is that sex is a natural soporific (that means sleepy maker) so slip the stripper heels back on her if they'll fit and bang away. Be gentle though, remember her haemorrhoids.

8.   Rib Pain

This is most common in the third trimester and is caused by Her uterus pressing into her abdomen and also wee Rocky punching the crap out of Her from the inside. This pain is usually felt on Her right side and is more painful sitting down.

How you can help:
Make sure she wears loose fitting clothing (to be honest. By the third trimester She really won't suit hot pants and bustiers). Make sure that she has plenty of pillows and cushions when she's lying down so that she can adjust them to find the best position. If the pain is severe She can try this exercise. Get her to stand around eighteen inches from a wall facing it (like she could stand any closer) and get her to cross her arms in front of her face. Next she leans her arms onto the wall and pushes them as high up the wall as she comfortably can. This should stretch out the diaphragm and ribs causing immediate relief. The good news is that the pain usually goes away once the baby has dropped into the pelvic area in preparation for birth.

9.   Sore/Tender Breasts

Now it's getting serious. Any threat to the boobies is a direct threat to our day to day pleasures. It is actually one of the very first signs of pregnancy. This tenderness commonly continues throughout pregnancy as the breasts enlarge, the milk ducts grow and stretch and the breasts fill with milk.

How you can help:
Stay away from them. Seriously, resist the urge to grab a couple of handfuls whenever she's standing at the sink. Check with her first. They won't always be too sore to touch and whatever she says be gentle with them. Also, and I don't mean to freak you out again but I told you that they can leak. You can also encourage her to get fitted for a more supportive bra. (You know the type. It tells her she's great and that she looks beautiful also that she's right, Susan at work is a cow. Now that's supportive. Badoom tish) Buy her a multivitamin specifically designed for pregnant women and get her to take a vitamin B6 supplement in conjunction.

10. Thrush

Candida Albicans is not the name of a stripper despite how apt a name that would be. It is actually the name of the fungus which causes thrush. This organism lives quite happily in the intestines of both men and women but one third of women also have it present in their vagina. During pregnancy the vagina becomes rich in glycogen which is a form of glucose. This feeds the fungus. This is part of the reason that pregnant women are 10 times more likely to develop thrush. A simple analogy is this. A non pregnant woman's vagina is like a youth hostel to thrush If it's on a budget backpacking around Europe's vaginas whereas a pregnant woman's one is a five star resort in Monte Carlo paid for by the wealthy yet still hot widow who picked it up hitchhiking. In other words there is a pretty good chance she will develop thrush so it's best you know the symptoms no matter how gross they are. Let's start with the thick, white cottage cheese-like discharge from her vagina. (I wasn't kidding about the gross part.) This is usually accompanied by intense itching, vaginal dryness and a burning sensation while having sex or urinating. By the way, it's catching so resist the urge to have sex. Try shoving it into a pot of cottage cheese. It's as near as damn it to the real thing I understand.

How you can help:
Get her a supply of probiotic yoghurt and garlic also helps apparently (It should also keep vampires away). Check with her doctor for treatments and seriously, she may be embarrassed by this whole thing so try to be as supportive as possible. Like so

much to do with pregnancy, save it up for giggles after the baby is born.

11.   Varicose Veins

Varicose veins are swollen, twisted veins usually in the legs but sometimes the anus (good old haemorrhoids) or vulva. They are a common ailment during pregnancy as a result of rising blood pressure in the legs. This is caused by the enlarged uterus interfering with the blood flow between the legs and the heart. There is no great risk with varicose veins but they are unattractive and may cause stress to her already overburdened ego.

How you can help:
Encourage her to keep the weight off her feet as much as possible and to keep her feet raised on a footstool when possible. While she's sitting encourage her to make fists with her toes, circles with her feet etc. massage can be used as a preventative measure but if she already has them do not massage the area. Support stockings and flat soled shoes can also help. Flat shoes and support socks? I think I've just found the only fetish that doesn't exist on the internet.

So, there you have my personal top eleven pregnancy ailments. Why eleven? Why not? Anyone can have a top ten or dirty dozen. It takes an artist to have a top eleven. Mark my words. I'll be famous for top eleven lists one day. Anyway, the list above while comprehensive is not complete. She may experience some of, all of or more than these throughout the forty weeks and you won't so give her all the help, support and love you can. Remember one immutable and oh so important fact. She is a woman and as such has all the body insecurities that even the most flawless Playboy centrefold has. Take those insecurities and then cover the legs with veins and have haemorrhoids coming out of her arse while cottage cheese and god knows what else is coming out of her vagina and you have the recipe for a very unhappy woman. Help her wherever you can and constantly reassure her that She's beautiful and you love her. Everything in the list above is temporary or treatable so tell her there's light at the end of the vulva. Even if you literally dry heave every time she steps out of the shower. Hide it and never,

ever let her know you ever felt like that. Unless you're having an argument. Then throw her ailments right into her swollen face.

That's a joke. Never tell her. She'll know but she'll love you for lying.

Top Five Inappropriate Songs to Play During Labour

1. "Three times a lady" by The Commadores
2. "I like big butts" by Sir Mixalot
3. "I've had the time of my life" by Bill Medley & Jennifer Warnes
4. "It's the end of the world as we know it" by REM
5. "Fat bottomed girls" by Queen

What complications can there be?

You name it. I don't mean to be flippant here but there are myriad things which can go wrong. I will deal with the truly awful such as miscarriage and cot death later and we've just spoken about the minor albeit annoying and embarrassing ailments she can expect so I think we need a wee bit of time to relax. Lets talk about something we really worry about.

Is it safe to have sex?

Simple answer is yes. Completely and utterly, one hundred percent safe. Unless of course She's married to someone else or She lives in the sea but otherwise, no risk at all. Despite what you may think, you are not long enough to give the baby a black eye or stab it or anything so don't worry on that score. Whether you'll want to have sex or not is another matter entirely. One friend of mine was genuinely freaked out by the thought of having sex with his wife from the moment he found out she was expecting. He actually said to her that he had always wanted a threesome just not like that, he'd hoped to ask her best friend. We never found his body but I'm sure the expression on his face would make a CSI investigator puke.

Seriously though there are a number of things which may freak you out. Let's get a few things out of the way though, to alleviate some of the more common fears. The baby will not feel, hear or see anything no matter which position you try. You can be on top without fear of crushing the baby although I recommend doggy style as she can continue eating while you do it.

You may continue to call each other any names you wish and talk as dirty as you like because the baby can't hear you and even if it could how is it supposed to know what "Ride me like a frisky piebald" actually means. I am so sure that your child can't understand what you're saying that I'll make a wager with you. If your kid's first words are "Fuck me harder" then I'll refund you the cost of this book.

As I mentioned earlier, the Booby Fairy arrives and gives you a wonderful gift at around three or four months. If you are especially lucky she will be over her morning sickness and the boobs won't be tender and she will be feeling hornier than a field of cattle (Horns - get it?).

If she is then go and frolic in the garden because, like a solar eclipse, the conditions need to be just right and it never lasts long. As pregnancy progresses she is going to feel more tired and emotional and may feel bad about her body and about as sexy as white slip on loafers on a man. She may not want anything to do with sex and if that's the case then go dig out your porn stash whenever Sleepy arrives for a visit and leave her alone. She will definitely want to have sex with you if she goes over her due date by more than a few days.

Apparently having sex is one of the best ways to induce labour. Maybe it's the rocking motion. Maybe the baby comes out to complain about all the noise. Who knows? The important thing is you get laid and however horny you are it's going to be a long time before you get any more. There is always a chance that you will be completely turned off by your wife's pregnant body. Some guys find a pregnant woman incredibly sexy while others feel that they would rather slam their dick in the car door.

Whichever way you feel is okay. If it is that you don't want sex then come up with a great excuse. Saying, I would but from behind it's like trying to tip over a cow and from the front I'm afraid your boobs will squirt me, will never go down well. You could try being open and honest about your feelings but how the hell do we do that? Saying that you are freaked out that you might hurt her or the baby is usually the best option. This makes you come across as caring and sensitive when in actuality you once saw two rhinos shagging on the Discovery Channel and you know you won't be able to get the image out of your mind.

Baby Bucket List:

We're all familiar with bucket lists. Loads of people make them. If you don't know what they are, a bucket list is a list you make of things you want to do before you die. Or before you turn 30 or 40 or 50. You get the idea. In essence it's a long list of things you can cry about on your deathbed as you realise you've only done two of them, and one of those was by accident. You have failed at life and now the grave beckons and you've never swam with dolphins or some shite. In actuality you've wasted your life and now it's too late. Cheerful stuff huh?

That's why I'm suggesting a Baby Bucket List. Much more achievable. You've only got a few months before B-Day (Do you like what I've done there) so lets make the most of it. Here to get you started is my own list
    Change your name.
    Emigrate.
    Have a vasectomy
    Start a new life as Senor Ricardo Montoya.
    Forget the last thirty years.

See how great that is? If you complete these steps I promise you all your baby worries will be over. I just heard from my editor and he says to disregard the previous list and may I just say that I will be taking everything seriously from now on. No more silliness.

Gotcha!

Actual Bucket List:

Go to the movies and watch a violent action movie. Once you're paying a babysitter you'll want to go drinking, believe me. You have the next ten years of animated toys, cars and aliens to look forward to. Some of them are great but there's very little chance of nudity.

Go afternoon drinking. I know you regularly go down to the local on a weekend afternoon for one and end up staying there for nine hours living on bacon fries and beer but you can't do that with baby. They never buy a round and they hog the snacks. Enjoy the lack of responsibility while you can.

Spend the day in bed. Literally. One Sunday you simply don't get up. Have the TV (Or iPad if you're fancy) at the bottom of the bed with some great box sets at the ready. Have your favourite unhealthy easy to grab food available and alternate between snoozing and eating. Do this for the entire day. It is allowed though not essential for you to get out of bed to use the toilet. On second thoughts, it is essential. No plastic bottle/bin liner toileting solutions please. Enjoy every second.

Go away with your mates. I don't care what your recreation de jour is. Be it golf, shooting, theatre or strippers and booze. Grab your mates and head off. You get a stag do before your wedding so why not have one before the baby. If you have a girl you may want to name her after a particularly beguiling stripper you met. (I know a guy who named his daughter Cherokee. When he told me I just took him over to my laptop, went to a random porn site and wrote that name into the search engine. We haven't spoken since. No loss, the guy was a dick).

Turn your TV and stereo up to the max and run around the house screaming at the top of your lungs while banging two pots together. Enjoy making noise now because soon you will travel everywhere like Tom Cruise in Mission Impossible. On guy wires and terrified of making the slightest sound in case the enemy wakes and all is lost.

Things to do with Preggo No. 3

Encourage Her to dress up one of Her friends in Her pregnancy jeans and then take them shoplifting. You could fit a frozen turkey up there. Think of the Christmas savings.

Male Sympathetic Pregnancy is a myth, right?

Male sympathetic pregnancy, also known as Couvades' Syndrome, also known as Big Girls Blouse Disease is not a myth. The title male sympathetic pregnancy comes from women's magazines to show the sensitive side of men. The term Couvades' Syndrome comes from the French word couvee meaning to hatch and shows that the French do actually have a sense of humour. The final term is my own because I am a dick. BGBD is not a myth. There are some men out there who experience weight gain, morning sickness and abdominal pain along with their partner. Come on. I experience that most weekend mornings. If you are one of the few unfortunates who suffer from this terrible affliction. Take heart. There is a cure. Apparently once the woman gives birth the symptoms disappear. Or you could always have a hysterectomy.

Stevie's month by month guide to the creature inside her: 5th month

Your baby is now around half its birth size and jumping around like a gymnast on speed at times. It can even do somersaults. It can also hear certain things from outside so keep the swearing to a minimum. Freaky fact, if it's a boy its testicles have started to descend from the abdomen to the scrotum. Go on little guys... you can do it. Go Team Testes.

How the hell am I supposed to look after a baby?

Don't panic. Okay, don't panic any more than you already have been. Taking care of babies is not easy but it isn't rocket science either. You may think that you know nothing about babies and how to take care of them but you'd be surprised what you already do know. You know which end the food goes in and which end the poop comes out right? If you don't then you better learn. Shoving the bottle in the wrong end can only scar the little bugger for life. You know that the soft spot on top of the baby's head is actually its brain. Resist the urge to start poking it to see what baby can do. The image of a baby doing the can-can on the couch is hilarious but you're bound to poke too hard and it'll grow up to be a racist or something. Unless you want it to grow up to be a racist in which case your kid's fucked regardless.

Here's my advice. Get someone's baby. I'd highly recommend that you ask their permission first. But get someone's baby and practice with it. Not soccer practice. Keepy uppy is a definite no no.
Seriously though. If you can get access to a sibling's baby for an overnight you can learn lots before the pressure of your own baby comes along. I can't stress enough to borrow a good baby. Grabbing your brother's colicky nightmare is a sure fire recipe for terrifying you both as to what might be looming around the corner. If possible, borrow a well behaved baby and take care of it for twenty four hours. Believe me, its parents will love you for it and best of all the obligation of reciprocation will mean that you can guilt them into doing the same for you when your baby arrives.

Now, parent the shit out of that baby. Feed it, change it, bathe it, dress it, sing to it. Basically everything you're going to be doing with your own baby. Before the birth of my first son I had not changed a nappy in eighteen years. It is definitely not like riding a bike. You do forget how to do it. Also you shouldn't wear those spandex romper suits cyclists wear either. Once you've had a bit of practice you'll realise that She is way more interested than you are when it comes to bathing, dressing and feeding the little treasure. Encourage this. Ultimately this means you'll have less work to do when your own bundle comes along.

In all seriousness. I completely understand that you're freaked out about at the thought of actually being responsible for a tiny helpless creature. Now you know how Papa Smurf felt and he had 99 of the little blue bastards to take care of. That and the fact there was only one female smurf must have led to tension. Not least tension in the smurf department if you know what I mean. Alright, I promised to be serious and I went off on a tangent of soft core smurf porn. (a sentence I'm pretty sure has never been put in print). Sorry, the reason I'm being so flippant is that I know you're scared and nothing I say will change that. Try to take comfort in the knowledge however that every new parent goes through these exact same fears and we still somehow manage it. So will you.

Top Five Tricks to Play on Her

1. Whenever She backs up, make truck reversing beeping noises.
2. If you're sitting on one end of the couch and She comes in and sits on the other, leap up the moment She sits down as if you've been catapulted into the air.
3. Tie a boomerang to the strap of her robe to help her put it on
4. Buy three pairs of shoes. One in her size and one each a size higher and lower. Swop around the shoes as often as you like. She'll think her feet have gone mad
5. Record Her late night fart noises and when you have enough, make a playlist of the loudest ones. Play it whenever friends come around so they can share in the pregnancy too.

What sort of dad will I be?

I really can't answer that for you dude. Even you probably can't. No one knows for sure just how good or bad a father they will be but what I can help you with is to point out the sort of dad you should avoid like the plague. Not just avoid becoming, avoid coming into contact with at all. I am pretty sure you'll never be like these guys purely because you've had the excellent taste to read this book (and any other subsequent titles by the same author) but also because you're not a complete dick. I know I'm speculating here but you're not are you? Good, assumptions made, we can move on.

I am going to run through some of the types of daddy you'll come across. With a little luck and through no small thanks to me you'll have the benefit of early detection so that you can keep your interactions with these assholes to a minimum or better yet, avoid them altogether. Let's begin with some of the easier to spot ones.

First we have the "I'm too cool to be a dad" dad and he is one of the easiest to spot. He's the one in shades at a play centre, sipping a latte and reading a lads mag. He is impeccably dressed and painfully endeavours to make it look as though he's not a dad. What makes this even weirder is that they never realise that if we believe that they're not a dad then why the hell are they sitting in a play centre? This guy never embraced having a child. He's probably desperately immature and surely sulks whenever the baby cries while he's playing Call of Duty. How does a dad like this get his comeuppance? In two ways, the first is when his child pukes all over his brand new shirt just before a night out with the lads (lads in this case are guys in their late thirties who still go to nightclubs). The second is when his daughter grows up to be a stripper and his son grows up to be just like him.

Next we have the "I wish I could breast feed" dad. These are the dads who embrace fatherhood so hard that they somehow compress their testicles into some form of rudimentary ovaries. This decrease in testosterone leads to some radical changes. For one thing they commonly grow breasts. Not big fun ones that they can play with, just enough breast tissue to make it strangely hypnotic as they run towards you. They are stay at home dads who imagine coffee mornings with the gals rather than a threesome. They spend their days hovering around their offspring and empathising with the other mums. So, how does a dad like this get his comeuppance? In two ways, the first is when he comes home to find his wife in bed with another man and secondly, when his daughter becomes a stripper.

The next father to avoid is the organic dad. These are guys, almost exclusively middle class, who insist that every morsel of food that enters their child's mouth can be sourced back to the first drop of rain that fell on it and has only been fertilised by a mixture of environmentally sound compost and angels tears. These guys stare at the jar of ready made baby food you're attempting to shove into your squirming child's mouth as if it was a mixture of razor blades and curare (a poison found in the Amazon which was really popular in spy movies in the seventies but is now, sadly, out of fashion. Bring back curare, I say, let's start a campaign.) They will happily lecture you for hours on the importance of nutrition for brain development and how tap water causes autism and ADHD. How do these dads get their comeuppance? In two ways, firstly their kids go crazy for junk food when they finally get a chance to and end up living in a trailer gradually getting fatter until they become the focus of a daytime TV special where they have to tear down a wall just to get them out. Secondly, is when his daughter becomes a stripper.

The last of these dads I want to mention here is the "I'm a winner and so is my kid" dad. This guy is usually a sports fanatic but also one of those annoyingly upbeat arseholes who does two hundred sit-ups and goes for a five mile run before breakfast. They had a pushy father and by god they're going to push now. A simple egg and spoon race has them practicing for weeks with their child. Racing around a frosty field at dawn and experimenting with various types of eggs. These dads will only make you feel bad about your beer gut and the fact that your own kid ate the egg and then fell over at last years sports day. How do these dads get their comeuppance? In two ways, firstly when their kids grow up to be equally competitive, even to the point where it's a point of pride to get dad cheapest nursing home possible and secondly, well do I have to say? You get it by now.

I know that I've used the example of a man's daughter becoming a stripper as some sort of bad thing and let's be totally honest here. It is a bad thing. Which would you rather? A daughter who can go up a pole faster than a fireman can come down it or a daughter who can perform the open heart surgery you're bound to need some day? See, I'm a big fan of strippers. I think they do a hell of a job but would I want my kids to be one? No way. Not least because they're boys.

In all seriousness. You are going to meet a lot of new men once your child is born. From religious ceremonies to birthday parties and from school runs to trips to A&E you will meet dads wherever you go. The vast, vast majority of them are just like you. They love their kids, they're afraid of Her and they are desperately hoping that you're not a dick. You might even make some new friends and be organising play-dates for yourself before long. You should use this parenting lark as a way to meet other like minded guys who can help you to recognise and avoid these dads we spoke of. Remember, they are hoping, as you are, that you're not a dick. So don't be.

What exactly are Ante-natal classes and do I have to go?

Can you imagine anything more horrifying than spending your hard earned evenings and the occasional Saturday cooped up in a room with a load of pregnant women, a lesser number of pissed off fathers-to-be and one tampon rolling Earth Mother? Well, you will. Now, add to that the overpowering stench of ylang ylang cloying at your throat and the gentle sounds of pan pipes in your ears while Mother Nature leads all of you in a mass breathe in (and out obviously). You'll sit there, cross legged on a cushion on the floor silently contemplating the consequences of standing up and shouting Fuck it. I don't care if the fucking kid never comes out.

Don't worry. What you're feeling is perfectly normal. While it isn't easy hang in there, you've accepted so much so far. The changes in Her, the constant ever-changing demands, having to appear interested whenever she pulls out the baby book. But this is a step too far. You feel ridiculous, you're bored out of your mind and the collected noises of adenoidal breathing and pregnant farts have finally pushed you over the edge.

Bad news dude. However bored you're feeling is irrelevant. She loves this shit. She is surrounded by other like minded (that is to say; mental) women with a common goal and common complaints. So, suck it up and sit there trying to look interested. To help you pass the time there are a number of games you can play. Play the "what size was she before?" game. This is where you pick out a woman at random and try to guess what size she used to be. Ten points for boobs, twenty for arse. You get the idea. Or why not play the "which dad is having an affair?" game. This is self explanatory and does make you feel better about your fidelity. Make up back stories for all the people there. Which dad doesn't know that he's not the father? Which woman has been sneaking nips of breast milk when no one is looking? I imagined that the Earth Mother was actually a disgraced nurse who had to quit due to the inordinate amount of patients who died while she was on shift.

I think it's pretty obvious that I didn't pay much attention during the ante-natal classes. I get bored easily and have a vivid imagination. Normally I'd picture all the women in the room naked but that wasn't an option this time obviously so I was left with my serial killer/lactation fetishist fantasies. (That previous sentence sounds like something you'd hear read out by a psychologist in court doesn't it?). The thing is though; I should have paid more attention. At least to the breathing exercises. These really help Her during labour and as She'll be a little distracted it's a real help if you know what you're doing and so can help her to focus. I just realised that I used the word help three times in the last sentence. Now, that either means that this is really important, or that my subconscious is screaming and I need to get medicated.

Okay, here's the grown up part. The ante-natal classes are a real help to Her. It's where She can get the answers to all those questions you're too disinterested to care about. (She's a woman. There's no limit to the number of questions.) She will have a genuine, bona fide expert there to offer advice and support at a time when She is really beginning to realise She's actually going to have a baby. The impending birth is becoming more and more real to her and her anxiety levels are increasing. Being in a supportive environment is great for her if a bore fest for you. Sit back, admire the boobs and pay attention when the subject of breathing comes up.

There are a few things you, as her ever vigilant protector, need to watch out for however. Firstly, be aware that they may show a graphic video recording of someone giving birth. Ask if they will show the extended directors cut preferably with commentary. Check with Her before the class and make sure that she's comfortable watching it. If she's happy then buy some popcorn and sit back.

Alternatively, She may not want to see it and if so skip that class or part thereof. The Earth Mother may try to encourage her to watch it "to help prepare" Her for labour. If this happens threaten to set fire to her dream catcher and run away. Bottom line is that if She doesn't want to watch it then there's no one on earth who's going to make her. If you want a great laugh force the women there to watch the birth on shuttle search rewind. The moment the baby shoots back in should be priceless.

While some classes really do have an Earth Mother type the majority are run by nurses or midwives who are founts of information. The other thing to be aware of is that despite their qualifications some of these women will be shite. Some will want to regale the women with birth horror stories or cajole them into natural births. Your job is to keep an eye out for these, albeit rare, types and take them out if necessary. So, to recap. Antenatal classes are great, except when they aren't and you have three simple jobs. Firstly, find out if there's going to be a gore filled video nasty and check if She's okay to watch it. Secondly, make sure the facilitator isn't some attention seeking doom merchant and if she is make sure it's a double tap to the head and finally and most importantly; Learn all the breathing exercises and practice them so that when the time comes you won't be standing there gasping like a fish in a rowboat. Easy.

What advice do you have on being a father?

Tell your wife you are having problems with your hearing and buy a hearing aid about 3 months before birth. Wear it around the house and particularly around bed time. At night time always make sure to take it out. Always make sure to make comment about taking it out. Try to make a joke out of it, for example: "Goodnight love, you can snore all your want because I won't hear a thing", "Love you dear, you better respond quickly because I'm taking my hearing aid out" etc. When the baby is born continue as normal...

Ian, CEO

Breathing Techniques in Labour ·

Learn the breathing techniques yourself so that you can help her during labour. Here is a back of a beer mat guide to what She should do and how you can help.

She should not hold her breath, which we do when taking a large crap, this leads to her expelling too much air and gasping afterwards which can lead to her hyperventilating. The most important aspect of these breathing exercises is that she concentrates on breathing and not the pain. It is important that her breaths are shallow as she does not want to breathe deeply into her abdomen. After all, that's where the pain is.

There is also the Huffing and Puffing technique where the emphasis is on the exhale: blowing as if you were trying to blow the candles out on a birthday cake. Practice these a few times a day. Always emphasise the outward breath. No blow job jokes please. For once in her life she won't be in the mood to talk during contractions so answer for her if you can and tell people to wait if you can't. Get her to focus on some spot to help her concentrate: a picture, a piece of equipment or your crotch. Its part of the reason she's here in the first place. Seriously though, learn these techniques and practice them often. It will make a huge difference in her pain management.

Chapter 4

Foetuses and Ferraris

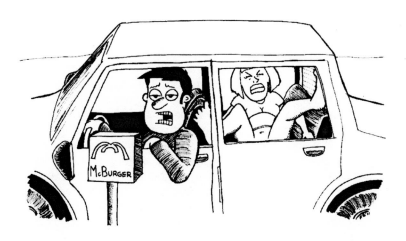

"So that's one super size meal and, What are you having love?"

Why are they showing Me Pictures of an Octopus?

The first time that the pregnancy becomes "real" for a lot of couples is when they go for the first ultrasound scan. It usually occurs in or around the third month and it is pretty amazing. You get to see the tiny heart fluttering away and you are aware that this life was created from the love you both share...

Are you alone? Are you sure? Okay, good. The whole scan thing is weird. First they cover her bump in KY and then run a supermarket pricing gun over it. I kept waiting to hear that familiar beep noise and then find out that my kid was on some form of buy one get one free special offer. Yes, you get to see the heart fluttering away but once you see that it's working fine and that the baby is alive and well then you start to look around the screen, searching for that most desirous of appendages, the wee willie.

I know that we have to say that we don't care what sex the baby is so long as it's healthy but come on. This is a book for men; we're not here to bullshit each other. You want a boy. Not least for the reason that you know way better than her just how truly awful men really are. There's no way you'd want to bring a little girl into this world. A sweet wholesome girl who then went on to meet a freak like you. Men are pigs, end of story. Now, it doesn't matter that we are nice and caring on the surface. When we are horny we're pigs and men are always horny. So, while we'll love the child no matter what the sex we want a boy at least first so that we can teach him to beat the shit out of anyone who comes on to his sister.

So you desperately peer at the screen looking for a nice, easily spotted little dinky waving away at you from its little amniotic bath. The bad news is that you won't be able to see it. All you'll be able to see is this gigantic eye which makes the whole foetus look exactly like an octopus. Great, you think, She had an affair with an octopus. Why an octopus? Sure they're good with jars but so are you if someone dries it with a tea towel first and maybe loosens it a bit for you. (that is a reference to a little known fact about octopi which is probably the cleverest thing I've written in this whole book. Says a lot about the quality of the writing doesn't it?). They will even give you a photo of the little cephalopod (Seriously, how much are you learning about octopi today? This book just keeps on giving) to take home with you. This is a picture which is identical to every other scan picture taken since scans were invented. If you don't believe me ask to see someone else's pic. I guarantee you it will be the same as yours. I think that they just print out the same one over and over again to save money. Just pretend that it's really special.

In all seriousness the first scan really is a big deal. It really does bring it on home to you and hearing that racing heartbeat for the first time affects every man. Whether you feel love, responsibility or some sort of flashback to going clubbing in the nineties you will feel different when you leave after hearing it. She will probably by way more gooey about the whole thing but be aware that She may be completely freaked out as well. As I said earlier, this makes everything seem more real for both of you. She may now experience the crashing realisation that there's a baby inside her that's going to have to come out at some stage. She may not initially be all sunshine and roses about the whole thing but that's completely normal too. She will probably feel that there's something wrong with her if She doesn't immediately bond with it. There isn't and this is very common. Let her react however She chooses and be there for Her to talk. Let Her know just how common it is for a woman to be weirded out by the first scan and that there's nothing wrong with Her reaction. However She's acting, as usual be supportive. Say positive things like "It's going to be strong, look at those legs" or compliments like "It has your eye". She won't care. She now has proof positive that there's a wee baby growing inside her and in time or straight away She'll fall in love with Octobaby and be knitting eight legged babygrows in no time.

Stevie's month by month guide to the creature inside her: 6th month

Your baby is around 20cm long and has developed loads. It can kick, grasp and even react to bright light shone on its mother's stomach. Freaky fact: it's hiccupping a lot in there like some tiny belligerent drunk. Good news is, if the baby were to be born now it could survive with intensive care. Yay!

Hot wheels

Here is your moment. Finally, this whole pregnancy lark is paying off. It's buggy buying time. A time when all men's thoughts turn to space saving vs. weight saving and value for money vs. go faster stripes. Forget sterilisers and breast pumps. Not for you the changing table and baby bath. This is your domain. This is like buying a car for God's sake. This has wheels and a brake, albeit a rudimentary one.

I have a nugget of information for you. I know I shouldn't say but I have to. Are you sitting down? Good. Hold on to your hat because what I am about to tell you will finally bring this whole pregnancy deal to life for you. Here it is ...Ferrari make baby buggies!

I know! I know, Ferrari - as in the formula one/super car Ferraris. They make buggies, for babies. Now, before you get too excited let's get a few things clear. They do not have engines. I know, I too would love a four hundred and fifty brake horsepower buggy to fly around the shopping centre. I think it's pretty much essential. Think of it, the shopping done in a fraction of the time and all the honeys eyeing you up as you do so.

Come to think of it, it's irresponsible of Ferrari not to put an engine into one. Damn their Italian horsey hides. Still though, it is made by Ferrari and it has the logo and everything. At the end of the day you can still tell people that you own a Ferrari. There is one teeny wee downside which stupidly practical and rational people (such as you know who) may throw in your face: the fact that it damn near costs as much as a real Ferrari.

But it's a small price to pay to end up in a position to legitimately wear a Ferrari jacket to work. Tell her that they are the safest buggies on the market and that they have been proven to remove stretch marks when pushed. If that doesn't work, sulk; sulk like you have never sulked before. If necessary throw a full on hissy fit and play the "No one cares what I think, I'm just the dad" card. It probably won't work, but believe me, barring six wee balls with your numbers on them flashing across your Saturday night TV screen, this is the only chance you'll ever get of owning a Ferrari. By the way, if you do fail in your bid for a Ferrari buggy fear not, Porsche make them too.

Okay, once again it's time to be serious. There are only a few things to keep in mind when buying your buggy.

- Weight
- Ease of use
- Bulk

The weight issue is fairly self explanatory. Get the lightest one you can. It may seem obvious but in a world filled with cup holders and removable wheels all is not as simple or as light as it would appear. Remember you are going to need a travel system. (Great name huh?) A travel system consists of a pram which can be used as a buggy when the child gets older and a car seat which is, and rightly so, mandatory under the law. Yes, I know that It would probably fit in the glove compartment but then where would you put your gloves? Honestly, have you ever put gloves in your glove compartment? Know anyone who does? Of course not, this isn't the 1920's.

But as usual, I digress. These things weigh a tonne. Also, what you are putting into it is only going to increase in weight so be prepared for that. Pretty much every parent I know buys a lightweight buggy once the baby can hold it's head upright. The bulk is also a huge consideration. (When I say bulk, I don't mean Her). The boot of my car could easily hold three sets of golf clubs and enough beer to drown a small cow yet when I put the pram of our travel system in there its can only hold that and maybe have enough room for a small fart.

Finally there's ease of use. I have seen mechanical engineers reduced to quivering tearful wrecks trying to put up or down some of the buggies out there. Some of them are like some giant Rubik's cube which can only be used by someone with three arms, two of which are ambidextrous. It's common to have to pull two separate levers while pushing a pedal with your foot just to get it up and then just as you are about to put baby in, the whole thing snaps closed with the ferocity of some sort of giant mousetrap. All this while standing in a rainy car park in November.

Here's the simple advice. Go to a good, reputable baby shop and pester the shite out of the staff. Get them to explain everything and show you how it all works. Don't do the guy thing and nod sagely all the while marvelling at the size of some of the other customers boobs. Get hands on. Not with the boobs, pervert. Get hands on with the travel system you think you want. Lift it. Shake it. Put it up. Put it down. Stop sniggering at all the double entendres racing through you mind right now.

Get them to show you how to install the car seat. Now you try. Now get them to show you again. I can't stress the importance of this. Believe me, even after it's been installed, you are bound to have to move it to another car for a trip or take it out just to clean up the puke that's slid under it during some long, bumpy car ride. All joking aside. A badly installed car seat could kill your child. So, no excuses. Learn how to do it right. So, to sum up. Try to get the lightest, simplest and most space saving travel system you can afford.

I know, why not get the Ferrari?

What one piece of advice would you give to a man on how to handle his pregnant partner?

"With oven mitts at the end of a non conductive stick from 3-7 feet away depending on size and mobility."

Ross, Comedian

Why am I here?

Don't worry dude. There's plenty you can do to help. You're a guy and planning stuff is what you were born to do. There is so much surrounding pregnancy and childbirth that is out of your control so it really helps both you and Her if you can take care of what you can control. First let's look at the hospital bag. Every pregnancy book has a pretty comprehensive list of items for the hospital bag. In fact you really should have two. One for the labour ward and one for afterwards. The latter should be comprised of baby stuff and girlie stuff. For the baby make sure that the bag contains:

- Nappies (Thousands of them, okay, I'm exaggerating a tad but seriously, bring lots)
- Baby Shampoo

- Mitts (Newborns scratch the shit out of their faces and in five minutes can go from cutie pie to horror movie extra. Think of the photos.)
- Hats (Newborns can't regulate temperature well so for the first few days they have to wear a hat. Don't worry, it makes them look all "Gangsta" and cool.)
- Bottles of readymade formula and teats. (You may well be planning to breastfeed but for a million reasons sometimes that's not possible straight away. Think of your Boy Scout training, Be Prepared)
- Clothes (Lots of clothes, bodysuits etc, pack as much as you think you'll need and then treble it, you'll thank me later)
- A toy that you bought. (Two reasons for this: One, hospital cots are so bare and severe looking its nice to brighten up your new baby's environment and Two, there's no better feeling than buying your child's first ever toy, trust me on this.)

For Her you will need:
- Loads of underwear, including disposable panties (Eew, Gross)
- Breast pads
- Make up (She is going to have to meet all her family and friends and will want to look well. It's not going to work but don't tell her that)
- Tracksuit bottoms and baggy clothes. (She will want to hide every part of herself for a while. Let her. No belly tops or hot pants)
- Toiletries
- Slippers
- Magazines, books, Nintendo DS. (She won't get to look at them but it will amuse her visitors for a while).
- Mobile phone and charger. (Come on, it's impossible to get her to shut up when she has nothing important to talk about. Now that she has an excuse…)
- Camera and bucket loads of film if it's not digital. (you will end up with a hundred pictures of a baby that looks like every other new born in the history of the world. Your scan picture is more individual.)
- Goodies and treats for her. (She is going to be starving for the next twenty four hours after expending that much

energy. Don't rely on hospital food or vending machines, bring a supply of her favourite stuff and step back.)

Your bag of stuff for the labour ward is your chance to shine. You need to fill it with anything and everything that will offer her some measure of comfort during this insane time. Imagine you are a Navy S.E.A.L. and you have been captured by terrorists. You have been taken into a windowless basement with a chair bolted to the floor being the only furniture. There is a drain in the floor to make it easier for your captors to sluice out the blood after interrogating prisoners. You are handcuffed to this chair and tortured in ways which you never believed possible and are experiencing pain the likes of which you heretofore had only imagined. Now, what treats would make this experience a little more bearable? Put them in the bag.

I'm obviously taking the piss but I used an analogy I knew you'd understand. You are going to help her through an agonising time and what you pack in that bag can really help. Here are some of the things I know helped:

- Chewing gum and mints. (During pregnancy and especially labour a woman's sense of smell is heightened massively and the last thing she wants is your fetid breath wafting over her and adding to her misery)
- Chocolate bars and energy drinks. (These are actually for you. You have no idea how long labour will last and the last thing you need is to have your blood sugar crash just when she needs you the most. Eat often but discreetly or you might end up with a Mars Bar rammed up your ass)
- Water vapourisateur. (This is a can of compressed water which comes out in a fine mist when you spray it. This is unbelievably refreshing and comforting for her between contractions, especially if you fan her face afterwards.)
- Magazines etc. (there can be long periods of inactivity during the first stage of labour where some form of distraction is welcome.)
- Clothes to dress the baby in. (In the movies the baby is handed to the mother swaddled in a blanket where it remains until it's of school going age. In reality, a nurse will ask you for the baby's clothes and then take it away, hose it down and dress it.
- Music and player - you might like to burn a CD or create a play list of some of her favourite music to play during

labour. I'll never forget hearing a woman swear like a career soldier and abuse everyone who came near her while "Once, Twice Three Times A Lady" by The Commodores played over the hospital radio system.

Lastly… Anything else she wants. - don't question, just get it.

Stevie's month by month guide to the creature inside her: 7th month

Your baby is now getting fatter. It's letting itself go terribly. Kidding. It's building up fat stores for after the birth and its brain is now developing rapidly. Freaky fact: most of the hair that covered it is now gone except for on the back and shoulders. It now looks like a topless Turkish waiter.

Managing the in-laws.

Q: What's the difference between outlaws and in-laws?
A: Outlaws are wanted.

Let's be honest here. You fell in love with her not her family. At the end of the day, no matter how well you get on with them they're still her family, not yours. If you don't believe me: cheat on her. Then see how close you all are then. Okay, don't cheat on her but don't for a second think that you are as important to them as She is. So, now that I've shattered whatever tenuous bond you had with your in-laws let's look at some of the areas you need to be mindful of lest this whole house of cards come tumbling down.

The first thing to consider is who to tell about the impending new arrival first. My advice is very simple. Tell her parents first and then immediately hang up and tell yours. Now, here comes the clever bit. Tell each one that they are the first people you've told but to not let on as the others are a bit funny about stuff like that. Clever huh? Now they both feel that they are the most important and that you agree that the other grandparents are dicks. You may think that this is a bit unnecessary and that your parents and hers are rational, lovely people who couldn't care about such minor things. Wrong, wrong, wrong, wrong, wrong.

Grandparents are the single greatest boon to the new parents or the single greatest pain in your ass. You can't tell which one's you have until the baby is actually born. The grandparents can be broken down into three loose groups.

- The Helpers.
- The Interferers.
- The Dead.

The latter really don't have that much of an influence unless there is some supernatural element involved here in which case I would recommend crucifixes at the birth and remember to check the baby's head for sixes. (More than two sixes is cause for concern, ask Her if she's slept with any jackals recently). The first two are much more common so I'll deal with them here.

Braxton Hicks

Braxton hicks or false labour is also the name of an album by an independent rock band from Australia called Jedediah. You might want to mention this during labour. I'm sure everyone will be fascinated.

I will make the assumption that both of you have both sets of parents above ground. That's four grandparents - two of each. Are we all up to speed? Good. If it happens to be the first grandchild then stand back. You may be inundated with offers of baby stuff, furniture, babysitting the lot. If it is the seventeenth grandchild then don't be surprised if no one notices a child hanging off Her boob for a change.

If you are lucky you get the Helpers. These are great and should be exploited until they drop. Literally. The Helpers bring home-cooked meals when they visit, refuse to let you change a nappy or give a feed and offer the greatest gift of all with their babysitting services.

Helpers remember when you were a baby but back then they were too tired or too busy to appreciate babyhood. Now, they are retired, have loads of disposable income and thanks to dementia have forgotten just how big a pain in the ass babies really are. As I say: run them into the ground while you can because soon enough they'll get bored with the Little Angel straight from heaven or worse yet another sibling will give birth to a newer cuter bundle and you've lost your workforce. So make hay while the sun shines or however else you get your kicks these days and bring on Granny and Grandpa Helper.

The other type of grandparents are the Interferers. They too are quick, but quick to condemn rather than quick to help. The Interferers feel that they know way more than you and take every opportunity to belittle, berate and criticize everything you are doing with the baby. This leads to huge rows as the one whose parents they aren't (another one of those eye-straining sentences there) wants to kick them out on their ass while the one whose parents they are reverts to their childhood self and just takes all the abuse.

Whichever type of Grandparents you're working with be aware of one immutable fact. No matter how well your respective in-laws get on the second the baby comes into the world the rivalry begins. If you're smart you'll capitalise on this and start playing both sides against each other. "John and Ethel were here last week. Oh, it was great to see them. They arrived with a load of toys for the baby and a case of beer for me. Then they gave us a voucher for a spa weekend next month and they'll babysit for the whole three days. They really are the best" With luck and some imagination you should be able to retire in a couple of years.

Both sides will of course piss you off. Believe me, if either one feels like they were less important they will make your lives a misery. Every intra-family get together from now on will consist of the sulky parents sitting at one side of the room and the unbearably smug ones sitting at the other. They will sit as far apart as possible and are bound to start fighting once the drink starts flowing. So, lie to them both and save yourself the cost of remodelling your local bar after the christening.

The next and infinitely more difficult task is managing the grannies. I'm sure that you have the stereotypical image of the apple cheeked granny with an apron full of toffees and a lap full of knitting. Well done, you still exist in the 1950's. Today's granny may well have grown up in the seventies and partied in the eighties. That's the cocaine generation. Suddenly we know where granny's florid complexion came from. She may well have been snorting lines off a toilet seat when you or your wife was conceived so get the innocent granny image out of your mind right now.

Don't think granddad is all cardigans and slippers either. Thanks to the internet and Viagra there is every chance that he plays with himself more than you do. (Now we know why he spends so much time in the garden shed.) I'm not trying to shatter the image you have of your parents but I do want you to understand that grandparents are not what you think. They are just as human and as big assholes as we are and never forget that.

So that's where the main problem arises. Both grannies will believe that they know best and will have absolutely no problem vocalizing that. No matter how tempted you are never point out that it's been forty years since they looked after a baby and that things have changed. That will only lead to a lecture about giving birth while toiling in the fields and making nappies out of nettles. Just nod pleasantly, Bite your tongue and agree with whatever is being spouted at you. Why? Remember, grannies are the greatest source of cheap labour since the Indonesian baby boom. They will act as babysitters, child minders and even take the baby for weekends. This is worth more than anything and a bit of humble pie eating now is more than compensated for by the tequila drinking you can look forward to later.

As usual, it's time for a bit of seriousness. You may be lucky and have great in-laws and even greater parents who get on and only have both of your best interests at heart. If so, I'm delighted for you. There is a chance however that you have interfering busybodies for in-laws and complete dicks for parents. If so, you have my sympathies. You may have a combination of both. Okay, now that I covered all the bases here are a few things to be mindful of to ensure continuing babysitting without homicide attempts from either of you. Firstly, be aware that however they get on the grandmothers are women and as such will believe that they and they alone are right about everything to do with babies. If they have polar opposite views just agree with each of them when they are apart and keep changing the subject when they are together.

Keep an eye on Her and make sure that She's not being bullied by either her mother or yours. I know that sounds a little extreme but remember what I said in the beginning. You are not a true member of the other's family but thanks to genetics and recombinant DNA the baby is. So, granny can justify encouraging (i.e. bullying) Her because it's in the best interests of her grandchild. The simple rule of thumb is that you need to protect Her from your mother and protect yourself from Hers. Don't expect Her to do the fighting. Your mother will love you no matter what so there's no risk to your relationship with her while Her mother will hate you no matter what so there's no risk there either. The simplest thing to do is allow both sets of grandparents to spoil your baby and let them babysit as often as the wish. Then you and Her can go down the pub and bitch about them to your hearts content. While you're at it ask granddad to recommend some good porn sites and ask granny if her old cocaine dealer is still alive. It's a lot better than toffees and pipe tobacco.

Top Five Most Popular Male Porn Star Names

1. John
2. Ron
3. Nick
4. Adam
5. Steve (Yay for me!)

What's the hardest thing about babies?

Lack of sleep, lack of sleep and one more thing...lack of sleep. Without question the lack of sleep is the single hardest thing to deal with when it comes to babies. Sleep deprivation is banned by the Geneva Convention. It has been used to extract confessions and information for hundreds of years and there is no way to prepare your body for it. It is considered a cruel and unusual form of torture if you do it to a fundamentalist terrorist but if it happens to you because your baby has colic, no one cares.

The only way to get through the first few months of sleepless nights is with teamwork. You have to share the load. Even if you are the one back at work with the commute, the nine to five and the commute home again, you still need to help with the late nights. Of course, you are going to come home from work knackered and dreaming of an evening with your feet up watching the telly and yes, you even deserve it but remember, she has also been working all day and her boss is a cranky bastard all the time and lets face it. You never have to wipe your boss' arse for him. Kiss it maybe but never wipe it. So no, you won't be getting that night in front of 24 or The Sopranos you sorely crave. Just content yourself with buying the box set when it comes out.

As I have mentioned before, you have to be honest with each other. You are exhausted, is she even more so? If she is, it's up to you to take over. Do the next two feeds and let her recharge. Obviously the reverse has to also be true. If you are the most wasted one or if you have a career threatening presentation in the morning then you need to have the rest. With either scenario let it be understood that the favour will be reciprocated. It's also vital to let each other know when you are going to give the other a break. By this I mean, if, for example, you are going to do the next two feeds and look after the baby, tell your partner this in plenty of time so they can relish and look forward to it. It's a great help to be surprised with a lie in but it's even better to know when you fall into bed that the next two times the baby cries you can ignore it. Bliss, trust me.

Of course you are going to resent each other and there will be times when you both feel too exhausted to continue and are convinced you are the most tired. I feel a plain old fight to the death settles this particular scenario. Don't worry, if you are both as tired as you claim you won't be able to inflict any serious damage to each other. I have visited a cloistered order of silent monks, I have scuba dived thirty feet under the sea and I have even once experienced being in the eye of a hurricane but I have never experienced stillness and silence like the immobility two people can achieve when a baby cries at three in the morning.

You are both lying there. In the most potent battle of wills since Kennedy and Khrushchev during the Cuban Missile Crisis, you both know to move is to admit you are awake and therefore must get up with the baby. My only advice for this situation is to utilise your superior fantasy creating abilities. Sure, she may be able to imagine a slow dance with George Clooney on the deck of a yacht moored at Cannes for the film festival but you're a man damn it. You have spent your life fantasising about having sex with the most unattainable women and scoring the winning goal in the final when you are as unfit as your average internet blogger and about as attractive to women. Use that ability to completely lose yourself in make believe.

As you lie there with your baby roaring and your partner wondering how you can sleep through it all you have to do is imagine you are escaping from a team of highly trained baddies who are trying to get the microfilm you have secreted on the back of your eye patch. You are hiding in the woods as they search all around you but with your secret service training you know that you can remain motionless and undetected for hours if necessary.

See how easy that was. Now, when your wife gets up to tend to the baby you can go back to your fantasy about eight women forming an orderly queue beside your bed or whatever. Just remember to claim having heard nothing when you are quizzed the following day. There is some light at the end of the tunnel however. It won't last forever. The good news is that generally after around three months your child should be in some sort of routine and you may be able to catch a few zz's every few days or so. If you are especially lucky your baby may even start sleeping the night through at this stage. It's rare but not unheard of. Cling to that hope the same way that selfish cow Kate Winslet clung to that board at the end of Titanic. Come on, there was room for ten people on that plank but she let poor old Leonardo sink like a stone. You may be lucky and have that happen.

Different Birthing Options:

As with most things these days there are a number of choices for delivering the baby other than the traditional hospital route. Home births and water births are increasingly more common. A home birth is exactly like it sounds. She stays at home until labour begins and then you contact the birthing team.

I love that name - it puts you in mind of a group of maternity super heroes. One has huge hands like a baseball catcher's glove for when the baby shoots out. Another has super strength and can hold a pregnant woman's legs in the air for as long as it takes. Home births are ideal for women who have been through labour without complications before. As with anything there are risks but for some the benefits greatly outweigh them. Some women feel much more comfortable being in the hospital surrounded by professionals just in case something goes wrong.

Another option is a water birth. This can be done at the hospital or at home. If you choose a home water birth you arrange to have a birthing pool set up in your home for the birth. You can also have a water birth in some hospitals. Resist the urge to record the birth and title it Wet n' Wild 2: Pregnant Passion or some such. As with everything in life there are advantages and disadvantages.

Water births are increasingly more common but as with Home births there are always risks in the event of unexpected complications. Also, there is a chance for whatever reason that you both may be all geared up for a water birth and it's just not possible. Reasons such as: going into labour miles away from home, the water birthing suite being used by someone else or the birth progressing so quickly that the pool isn't full yet. There are any number of reasons why you may not be able to have a water birth as planned and this can cause quite a bit of stress for Her. You know what women are like when you change plans on them at the last minute. At the end of the day all both of you really care about is that the baby comes out and both She and the baby come through it safe and healthy. So whether She gives birth in a hospital bed, a birthing pool or while skydiving at 15,000 feet the most important thing is that someone catches It before it hits the ground. Here are the advantages and disadvantages of each type of birth.

Advantages of Water Birth to the woman:
- It is meant to be much less painful.
- The woman has much greater freedom of movement and therefore is much more comfortable.
- It can help keep the woman's blood pressure down.
- Water relaxes the pelvic floor muscles.
- It relieves anxiety and promotes relaxation.

Advantages of Water Birth to the man:
- It's a hot tub. Surely no one would mind if you had a dip afterwards.

- There's a chance the midwife will fall in - so many fantasies coming true.
- You won't have to shower that day.
- Constant hilarity as she's bound to fart a lot when she's pushing.

Disadvantages of Water Birth to the woman:
- Labour can take longer as contractions are relaxed.
- There is a risk of the baby getting an infection from the water.
- There is a slim chance of water embolism or drowning.
- The blood loss of the woman is considerable.
- The perineum softens which may lead to greater risk of tearing.

Disadvantages of Water Birth to the man.:
- No break immediately after the birth.
- If you're anything like me, all that water sloshing around will make you want to pee constantly (no pissing in the pool).
- Someone is going to have to clean up. She'll be tired and the baby's too young. Guess who's left?

Advantages of Home Birth to the woman:
- There is much less chance of MRSA and other infections.
- Everyone present at the birth will be known to Her unlike in hospital when pretty much anyone can wander by.
- Labour can progress normally without any interference.
- You can control the environment. Lighting, noise etc.
- There's no risk of travelling before the baby is born or bringing It home.

Advantages of Home Birth to the man:
- Your TV is there.
- Your fridge and your beer are there!
- Your golf clubs are within easy reach. You can pop out for a quick nine if you get bored.
- You won't have to pay for parking.
- Unlimited cups of tea/coffee/heroin.

Disadvantages of Home Birth to the woman:
- There is a greater risk if complications arise. i.e. emergency caesarean, forceps birth.

- It may not be covered by your health insurance.
- Analgesics and Anaesthesia may not be available.
- In an emergency: time is everything and transport may be difficult to arrange.

Disadvantages of Home Birth to the man:
- The mess. She'll probably be feeling a bit lazy after the birth so it'll be up to you.
- No break for you immediately after the birth so no strip club to wet the baby's head.
- Explaining to your neighbours what all the noise was about (Or don't. let them think you're hung like a mule.)
- It's gross.

> **How did you react when you heard you were going to be a father for the first time?**
>
> I was absolutely delighted....this was one of those rare occasions that was actually planned. It was amazing, scary and brilliant all rolled into one. I think I cried a bit.
>
> Daragh, Radio Presenter.

The Birth Plan

A birth plan is a great idea. It's basically a list that you make which outlines everything She wants from the birthing experience. Does she want soft lighting, minimal examinations, special music, a cocktail bar? Maybe not the last one but you get the idea. Sometime near Her due date the two of you should sit down and discuss how She would like the labour to go. Be aware that She may well be over sensitive to the baby's needs and ignore some of her own. This is another of those times where you can keep an eye on her decisions to make sure She's looking after herself. Having even a slight measure of control over the proceedings can help greatly with her feelings of helplessness. Your job is to carry a copy of that list with you and, as far as is humanly possible, make sure that the hospital staff adhere to her wishes. Of course some of the items on the list may not be possible but the odds are She'll be too busy to notice if one or two are missed. Whatever is possible is your responsibility. Forget your ego and embarrassment. This is one of your areas in which to shine so don't worry about the feelings or opinions of the hospital staff. There are only two people in that hospital you need to worry about: Her and the baby. You don't have to live with the staff.

Naming Your Baby

Naming a baby - what could be simpler? Here's my tip. Arrange with your lovely other half that if it's a girl she gets to name it and if it's a boy you get to. I know that sounds simple and rational but remember you are dealing with a hormonal psychopath who can turn on you with the speed of a cobra...on speed. Women should never be allowed to name a boy. They don't seem to grasp the concept of a decade of wedgies and cat calls aimed at an unfortunately named young boy.

My wife, who I adore, (I have to say that, trust me it saves a lot of grief) wanted to name our first child, wait for it...Felix. Can you imagine? Felix Cummins. That's feel, licks and cum all in the one name. He would be lucky to make it past junior infants. I would probably give him the odd wedgie myself. I wouldn't be able to help myself. Women choose names for boys that are cute. Forgetting the glaring fact that boys grow into men and saddling them with a name like Toby or Tarquin is practically assuring them a sex life that is entirely internet based. (Apologies to any Tobys or Tarquins who are reading this but you can't argue with me can you? You large forearmed creatures you. Come to think of it why would you be reading a pregnancy book? You were probably hoping for pictures of boobs.)

We should all have learned from celebrities by now that naming your child after an inanimate object or a season is not only wrong, it's borderline abusive. Do you think Peaches Geldof would be such a spoiled little cow if her name was Mary? I don't think so. So the following are out, despite what She may think; River, Summer, Apple (or any food for that matter), Moon-unit, IKEA or Kevin (I just don't like the name Kevin, Sorry Kevs).

Never name your child after a place name a la Brooklyn Beckham. I know he was named after the place he was conceived but if we all employed that rationale the world would be a much stranger place. Hi this is my son Boris, Boris in Ossery. Or worse, Hi, have you met my daughter? – "Back of a Ford Mondeo". Just get a baby name book and let fly.

Also, don't name your child Aaron. I know it's a nice name but it looks as though you read the first name in the baby book and couldn't be arsed going any further. Either that or you were too mean to even buy the book in the first place. Forget the meaning of the name too. It would be nice if our names meant "He who is super cool" or "hard ass motherfucker" but in reality a lot of names mean things like "bend in the river" or "peace".

> **Top five names to give your son if you want him to be beaten up:**
>
> 1. Rupert
> 2. Tarquin
> 3. Jeremy
> 4. Osama
> 5. Yoremum (Not a real name but just imagine the fun.)

Another good tip when deciding on what not to name your baby is to go for a drive through a dodgy area around teatime with the windows of your car open. It's an education I can tell you. All you can hear is a chorus of some of the worst names ever picked to saddle a child with or some of the most current TV character names.

When I was growing up there was an infestation of Scotts and Charlenes because of a particularly diabolical Aussie soap romance. Today there are a huge amount of Carries and Mirandas thanks to Sex and the City and I even know of a Wisteria named after the street in the TV show Desperate Housewives.

Also please be aware of what I call the "Jack and Katy Phenomenon". Quite simply, around eight or nine years ago everyone who was expecting a baby seemed to wake up on the same morning and decide to call their child Jack if it was a boy and Katy if it was a girl. If you want a laugh, go to any primary school at break time and yell out those two names. Honestly, it's like that scene from Spartacus.

"I'm Jack, no, I'm Jack."

Hilarious. Don't blame me if someone calls the police and you end up on a register however. And another thing: no matter how tempted you are never, ever, ever name your son after yourself. Nothing screams "I am self obsessed" like creating a clone of yourself. George Foreman, famous boxer and grill salesman has nine sons. Can you guess what he called each and every single unfortunate one? That's right. George.

Now that's just mental; and you aren't even famous. Who ever heard of Paddy McCarthy the fourth? So think hard brother. There is a family in Bedford in England, the Peacock family. Not the worst surname I can imagine. It's not great but it could be a lot worse. Ramsbottom for example, or Colon or Bin Laden. This would be a wholly unremarkable family but for the Christian name they chose for their son last year. They chose to name him Drew. Drew Peacock. Drew Peacock. Keep saying it aloud until you get it. Take your time. There you go. Holy crap! That kid is going to wander through life with the name Droopy Cock. But do you know what makes this such a cautionary tale his parents only realised their huge naming faux pas when the child had turned two months old. That means, he was baptised, registered and introduced to countless friends and family and through all that no one noticed that he was being named after Pele's medical affliction. (I don't know if Pele really has erectile dysfunction but he made that ad so now he's tarred with the same limp brush forever).

In Germany it is illegal to saddle your child with a name that may cause him ridicule or difficulty when he is older. I'm sure there are some civil libertarians out there who may feel a bit irked by this idea. Just to give you a prime example of this law in action. A few years ago a German family wanted to name their son Osama Bin Hitler. This was not permitted so they called him Fritz or Hans or something. I think they did the right thing. Naming your child is a huge responsibility. The name you pick now will stick with him like shit to a blanket - for eternity. If you are one of the unfortunate ones named Hubert or Emmanuel (two guys I grew up with, seriously) you get it. You know the pain of repeating your name in a nightclub as some girl cracks up. You've seen the smirk on the custom's official's face as he reads your passport. But the pain is not just for you alone. Think of your poor partner. Think of them having to tell their girlfriends that her new fellah's name is Rupert (I grew up with one of them too). Think of them having to cry out "Ride me, Humphrey" while in the throws of passion. Think of your children. Don't let it happen to them. You can break the cycle of abuse. I am quite happy with my name.

Steve. Steve's are cool. Steve's are the kind of guys who wouldn't get mad if you puked in their car. In fact they'd even buy you chips on the way home to replace the ones you lost. You've never met a bad Steve. Despite all that, I have laughed at enough names in my time and even watched as hundreds have done the same thing. Anyone who has ever been to a comedy club knows that the first thing we do is ask a few people in the front row what their name is.

You have no idea of the joy in a comedians heart when we hear a silly or pretentious name and realise we are going to spend the next five minutes taking the living piss out of you while everyone else in the room roars with laughter. Do you want that for your child? Do you want them to face that cringe worthy embarrassment? Of course not. So, as I say. Think hard brother and don't make the mistakes of so many others. Call them Steve (Stephanie if it's a girl).

What, if anything, would you have done differently during Pregnancy or Labour?

During pregnancy it might have been better if I had a job on an oil-rig or had joined the French Foreign Legion for a sojourn - anything to avoid getting in my wife's way! Alternatively I would liked to have been blessed with the patience of all the saints in heaven.

Tomas, University Lecturer

What major life changes should I make before it arrives?

The simple answer is none. Pregnancy is stressful enough without adding moving house or changing jobs into the mix. A lot of changes are headed your way so take your time and get used to some of them before you add more. Let's go through some of the major changes you'll have to make to accommodate the new arrival.

Firstly, I don't know what, if anything, you drive. If you already drive a large four door saloon car then move on to the next bit. You're covered here. If you ride a Low rider Harley or a Space Hopper, then things are going to change. At the very least you're going to have to grow up. Sure, nothing beats the rush hour commute better than a large orange ball with handles for ears and a sinister expression on its face but there is very little room for a baby seat on it.

Seriously though, you may well have to buy a new car, or at least new to you. At the very least you need a car with four doors and a huge boot. You need doors at the back because it's hard enough getting a baby in and out of the car at the best of times but trying to force a baby and car seat through that tiny gap where the seat folds down is something that wears thin really quickly. You also need an incredibly large boot. While the baby is tiny it comes with so many accessories that you almost need a trailer on the back. You may think that I'm exaggerating here but believe me, I'm not. The travel system alone should have its own postcode and add to that all the clothes, nappies, potions and unguents necessary for baby's hour-by-hour needs and you have a load that would kill a team of Sherpas.

Ideally a large transit van with padding on the inside is best. Just open the back doors, chuck in baby and all its various accoutrements and let them bounce around happily for the entire journey home. If you don't want to become a van driver than you'd better buy a large family four door saloon car with easily wiped down upholstery. I won't go into it here but the back seat of my car is an acre of stained material under a mountain of raisins, popcorn and Lego. Just get something big, safe and boring. You'll never regret it. (Except every time you get in or out of it, or when you're driving it, or when you're talking about it. Get used to the idea that your dreams of an Aston Martin DB9 are over.)

You may also have to move house to accommodate baby. Sure, it used to be great living in a studio flat with a 24 hour shop/chipper below and a discount drug dealer above but those will no longer be your major causes of concern after the baby arrives. You'll want more than one room not least because one of you will need to be sleeping while the other is feeding or changing baby and believe me that won't happen if the smell of poop and the sound of screaming invades your dreams. I imagine that's what causes serial killers to go on a spree. Their dreams filled with screaming and poop. You don't want either of you to become a serial killer do you? I thought not. So a new home is on the cards but unless your home is unhygienic or noise polluted then there's no reason to add the stress of moving on top of everything else until you've both had some time to become used to being parents. Give it a few months. When you do move you'll also have a much better idea of what the baby needs than you do now. For the first few months one of the greatest joys of parenthood is that the baby stays precisely where you left it. It can't walk, crawl or even turn over so you just need to ensure its environment is safe and hygienic only for around eighteen inches on either side of it. When it starts to move around then everything on the floor or within arms reach is food and nothing turns the stomach more than coming in to find your bundle of fluffiness eating out of the cat's litter tray. Sure their breath is fresher but it can't be good for them. So while they are immobile you can stay exactly where you are with breakfast rolls and heroin within a stones throw of your front door.

Things to do with Preggo No. 4

Use Her as an emergency seesaw when relatives arrive unexpectedly with their kids for a visit. Can also me used as a catapult in the event of unexpected Viking invasion. (You can never be too prepared).

Speaking of animals: some parents believe that pets can be dangerous around newborns and they can be, but some minor preparation and supervision should ensure that you don't have to abandon one family member in the woods just to accommodate another one. Also, the baby might end up being raised by squirrels and come to take bloody, acorny revenge many years later – which is my greatest fear. Treat your pet like you would treat your first child when a second one is coming. Reassure the pet with plenty of attention. Although you'll be pretty busy and focused on the baby, taking time to scratch it behind the ears every now and again, (the pet, not the baby, Idiot) may help guard against urine filled slippers every morning. Unless of course you have a drink problem or an especially bitter woman in your life, then piss drenched slippers are an occupational hazard.

So, there you have it. Yes you're going to have to make some pretty huge changes to your life and circumstances but there's no rush. As I said, take your time, get used to the new arrival and all the day to day life changes before you face the big ones. So climb aboard your Space hopper one last time, fill a syringe with grade A China White and bounce down to the 24 hour shop for some sweeties. Why? Because you're worth it.

What fun can I have?

I know it's hard to get interested in most of the purchases for the new arrival but there are a few gadgets that can help bring out your inner geek and allow you to have a little fun. I mentioned the travel system earlier and being a man I assume you have claimed this domain as your own. Let's see what other gadgets and gizmos are there to attract your beady eye.

First and foremost there is that essential bit of kit, the baby monitor. The array of features available on each model is staggering. You can have a one way communication system which allows you to hear what the baby is up to (i.e. ordering pizza or arranging a party with his buds). Then there is a two way system where you can communicate with it (i.e. telling him that you want extra pepperoni and that any party has to be over by midnight and no Wiggles sing-a-longs after ten). You can get monitors that light up in tune with your baby's noises. Like some sort of cool graphic equaliser. This is very handy when you have a load of people round for a party. The noise is bound to wake the baby and then all you have to do is turn off the lights, crank up the tunes and party. Who says having a baby eats into your social life?

I recommend the two way radio version as it gives you the chance to communicate with Her while She's tending to the baby. This is an excellent way of telling Her you need a fresh beer etc. without making Her have to come into the living room ons. See how caring and sensitive you can be when

... all seriousness, a baby monitor provides great peace of mind. There is nothing more reassuring than the sound of gentle snores wafting through that soft static hiss. It also means the little git is asleep and you finally have a moment's peace. I personally never had a use for a two way radio built into my monitor. It's advertised as a way to gently croon to your baby and lull them back to sleep without having to leave your armchair. Good luck with that. The only way I can imagine crooning a baby back to sleep with a few words is if I had somehow planted a post hypnotic suggestion into its wee brain and if I could do that I'd use it to make sure that It puts me in a decent nursing home when I'm seventy. Get one that has a battery pack or that has the capability to run on batteries. This means that you can be outside in the garden or in the strip club down the street and still keep an ear out for its needs. Never forget your responsibilities. That my motto.

Some monitors come with the technology to detect if the baby stops breathing and emits an alarm. You can also get mattress covers that perform the same function. If you want the extra peace of mind this brings feel free to get one. The last thing I would want is to discourage anyone from getting something which might protect a baby from harm but personally I never used one for two reasons. Firstly, with a baby monitor turned up high you can hear their digestive process so any change in breathing would be pretty apparent. The second and main reason I didn't is because a friend of mine had one for his baby and it regularly gave out false alarms giving my friend the most terrifying awakenings imaginable. Once when it was his turn to lie in his wife got up with the baby and forgot to turn off the monitor. In a moment of rebellion the monitor decided to wait an hour before noticing that there was no breathing coming from the long empty cot. The resulting siren caused my friend to leap out of bed convinced his baby was in jeopardy only to find that his baby had been abducted. His sleep addled brain couldn't deal with all this so he ran to the landing to search for his own private Lindbergh baby and promptly fell down the stairs breaking his leg. Now, I know that's a one off and the odds of that happening again are slim to none but I reasoned that having a baby was stressful enough without adding bone breakages and abject terror to the mix. As I say though. You can't put a price on peace of mind so feel free to get as technologically advanced a monitor as you can.

Sterilisers are a pain in the ass. They are essential, no question but the day you stop having to sterilise everything that's coming into contact with your baby is a real red letter day. This day usually arrives fairly soon after It starts crawling. Basically, once it starts crawling it will eat anything and everything it finds on the floor. For my first child we moved around in front of him scanning the floor for any speck of dust which might be destined for his mouth. For my youngest we called them floor snacks. I'll never forget the time that we found him sitting on the floor in our living room eating a hunk of bagel. We hadn't had bagels in a fortnight. See why we don't bother sterilising after that? It seems kind of pointless when the kid is eating two week old, hair and lint covered bread products to be concerned with the operational cleanliness of a bottle.

For my first son we used the old fashioned steriliser which basically works like a kettle. You wash and scrub everything, break it down into its component parts and then add a little water and switch on. The steriliser fills with steam and half an hour later you're left with half a dozen bottles a surgeon would be proud of. Now all you need is a hazmat suit and you can maintain sterility while filling them. For my second we used a microwave steriliser and this did the same job in a third of the time. There are really fancy ones, ones which use sterilising tablets, ones that rely solely on steam, even ones that use voodoo. You know the type. Place the bottles in Papa Shango's Super Steriliser, cut the head off a chicken, add the blood and some rum and away you go. Okay, I made up the last one. Not exactly hygienic but think of the drumsticks. Do a bit of research and get the one that sterilises the most bottles in the shortest amount of time with the least amount of chicken abuse possible.

There is a pretty cool gadget known as a Diaper Genie. (No it does not grant you three wishes or anything cool like that. If it did you'd only waste them. First wish; twelve hours uninterrupted sleep. Second wish; ten more. Third wish; that your kid's arse closes up.) Basically a Diaper Genie, or its equivalent, is a bin which you drop your foul smelling nappy into which then wraps it up in plastic and seals it and the noxious odour inside. It stores all these in a big long sausage-like bag for easy disposal. Most people agree that it works and really minimises the smell but at the end of the day the ass the poop is coming from is still floating around so don't expect this to ensure your home smells sweet all the time. There is also a cost element here as you have to buy refills for it but as you would have to buy nappy bags anyway it may not work out that much more expensive. In my not so humble opinion I wouldn't bother buying one. By all means get one if you are truly gadget obsessed but your home is going to smell of poop intermittently for the next three years or so regardless of what you do so you might as well just accept it. Training your child to use a litter tray might be the best option.

If you don't have a good camcorder and digital camera then now you have the perfect excuse to go and buy them. You will spend more time photographing, videoing and recording the minutiae of your child's life than you ever dreamed possible. You will have roughly five million photos of your first child and two or three of every subsequent child thereafter. If you are any sort of techno geek then there's no limit to the amount of editing and movie making you can enjoy. In actual fact, you'll get bored with filming the baby pretty quickly but She never will and while you're holding the camcorder you can't change the baby so feign interest and start rolling.

Speaking of all things geeky: if, like me, you have to work away from home at times a Skype subscription is great. No matter where in the world you are you can see, in real time, just how cute your wee progeny is and just how knackered She is. Nothing makes a hotel bed more comfortable than the knowledge that someone else is suffering. If you were in your own bed something would be waking you up every three hours demanding food, now you can just dial 0 and do the same.

These are just some of the many wee toys you can immerse yourself in just to make the whole baby lark more fun. From digital thermometers to automatic rocking machines, from bottle warmers to breast pumps the only limit is your imagination. Well, that and your bank balance.

How long was the longest ever recorded pregnancy?

The longest pregnancy recorded was 375 days. That's over a year for the chronically stupid of you. Over a year? The average pregnancy is 280 days. Can you imagine how pissed off She would be having to carry the baby for that long. Most women get twitchy if the baby is a day late, but three months. Wow. Personally, I can see the benefits of Her carrying it until it turns eighteen but then I've experienced the terrible twos. Weirdly, in this case the baby only weighed a little over six pounds at birth so at least if your missus does go over by a week or so you can reassure her that she doesn't have a toddler waiting in there. This incident happened in Los Angeles where baby Penny Diana Hunter was born to Mrs. Beulah Hunter after 375 days. I love that name Beulah. It puts me in mind of a beautiful Southern Belle. Although now it puts me in mind of a beautiful Southern Belle staggering around dragging her bump like one of those worlds strongest man contestants doing the Atlas Stones. I won't explain that last reference. You're men. I assume you know. If you don't go look it up.

You're welcome. Like so much of the information in this book keep that particular nugget to yourself. She doesn't need any more worries than she already has. Yes, it would be funny but seriously don't. Alright, go on then. Tell her.

There are of course suggested ways that you can kick-start the labour if Her due date is but a distant memory and there's still no sign of baby. The two most common ones are eating spicy food and having sex. Now tell me it wasn't a man who came up with that. "Uh, Honey. I read in a woman's magazine that the best way to induce labour is watch strippers while feeding your husband beer and chicken wings. Honestly, I saw it on Oprah too."

Nice one whoever came up with that? It gives me hope that we're not all weak willed kittens terrified of our women. I like to believe that there is a core group of men based in a volcano somewhere like The Justice League of Super Heroes. This group is the Justice League of Mankind. These are superheroes too but of a different kind. They are the ones who ensure that women don't completely take over. Like the French Resistance during World War 2. They are a ragtag group of ubermen. Men who don't just leave the toilet seat up. They rip it off altogether and shit in the sink. Real men. Men who use WD40 as a sexual lubricant. Men who didn't cry at Toy Story 3. Men we can only dream about being. They are the ones who came up with sex and curry as a labour inducer. They are the ones who keep the – guys sleeps with loads he's a stud/girl sleeps with loads she's a slut- social moray going. God forbid it was the other way round. These heroes transmit subliminal keep away messages into sports coverage which only affects the female brain so that we get some time to ourselves. It would explain why when women come near us while we're slouched on the couch watching football that they get so moody. God bless you Justice League. From all men everywhere: God bless you and take care on your perilous mission. Brings a wee tear to your eye doesn't it?

So, there you have it. There's always a chance that baby might decide to hang around for a while after the due date but if he does; think of it as a few more nights sleep for you and the chance of a curry and a shag to boot. There is of course the risk that this will prove highly effective and she may go into labour before you get a chance to finish. Good etiquette here demands that she at least gives you a handjob on the drive to the hospital. Some men don't want to risk the sudden contraction-death grip on penis hazard. This too is fine. In that case perhaps a quick bit of self pleasure as she's putting the hospital bags in the car. Sorry about that last. I think I'm still thinking about the Justice League. You put the bags in the car. She'll be ages getting dressed so you've plenty of time for self love.

There is however a second, more horrible scenario. There is always a chance that She could evacuate Her bowels during the later stages of labour. Now imagine a spicy Madras poo shooting out of her at the sacred moment a new life springs forth. What sort of a start in life is that? Forget the smell for a moment. Imagine you were recording the birth. I don't know if you're planning on recording the birth. You may have recorded the conception and would like to have the box set. Or, you may think that watching some blood and poo filled gore fest which quite frankly is much more fun to watch on rewind, is appalling. I know some people record it so that their kids can watch it when they're old enough. How old is that then? My guess is around NEVER years old. Dear God in heaven. The thought of my mother having sex appalled me since I became aware of the concept.

The thought of watching me come sliding out of her is second only to watching footage of me being conceived in my 101 things I never want to see list. Number eighteen is a sing-along screening of Mamma Mia so you know I'm serious. Some of you are now thinking surely there's no such thing. There is my friend; I've seen a herd of women leaving one such screening. I've never been more afraid in my life. If I looked even a tiny bit like Pierce Brosnan I wouldn't be here today.

What, if anything, would you have done differently during Pregnancy or Labour?

Both ours were born by emergency Caesarean section so I didn't have a great deal of time to dwell on anything. I was elated after they were born and couldn't understand why my wife didn't seem to share my joy, forgetting of course that she'd just had a serious operation. I was so mental I didn't cop on. My wife's biggest regret was torturing herself trying to get them to breastfeed when they just patently didn't want to. I think she felt very guilty about that.

Patrick, Comedian & Actor.

What do they mean she's going to be induced?

Inducing pregnancy is basically kick-starting the labour. While the majority of labours occur naturally there are times when it is deemed safer to induce labour rather than let nature take its course. If the labour goes beyond forty one weeks or if there is some risk to the mother or the baby by waiting, for example if She is diabetic or Her waters have broken but labour has not occurred. Certain conditions such as pre-eclampsia are grounds for induction also. Some women sometimes elect to have an induction if their partner will not be around for the birth. For example if the man is in the armed forces and is due to be stationed abroad before the due date an elective induction can be sought depending on time frames. If the father is in the armed forces he can point a gun at the bump and order the baby to come out with its hands up. This is usually very effective.

If the medical team and you both have agreed to an induction it usually follows a set pattern with some stages being tried a number of times before progressing to the next level. The first procedure tried is "Sweeping the Membranes" which couldn't sound more like a euphemism for masturbation to me. I was sweeping the membranes last night when I heard the front door open. I've never moved so quickly in my life. In reality this is where the doctor or midwife gently separates the membranes surrounding the baby during an internal examination. I'll be honest with you here. I have no idea what that means. All I do know is that it's very common, may be done a number of times and involves no medication whatsoever thus having no real risk to Her or the baby.

The next step is to use a pessary (like a suppository but for the front door if you follow me) or gel of a drug called Prostaglandin. This causes a slow release of the drug over 24 hours although it can be re-administered after six. The risks associated with this drug are small but they do exist. There is an outside chance that it can lead to overstimulation or hyperstimulation of the uterus. This can affect the oxygen getting to the baby. It's rare and the midwife will be very aware of it but as usual, keep your own beady eye open. If these methods do not work then a drug called Synctocinon can be administered. This is drip fed and really strong. Some women have complained of especially painful contractions while using this method and there also needs to be constant monitoring of the baby.

You may have heard of artificial rupture of the membrane or ARM. (Could they come up with a better acronym than ARM for something that's going to be shoved up inside Her?) This is where a device, not unlike a crochet hook (sorry, I forgot that you have no idea what a crochet hook looks like. You know the flat metal thingy that car thieves in the movies use to break into cars? Imagine a pointy one of them) which is used to rupture the membrane thus breaking the waters. This is rarely used on it's own as it isn't super effective and can leave the baby prone to infection.

Obviously, a naturally starting and progressing labour is desirable but if induction is necessary don't worry. The midwife will be keeping a close eye on things and at least you'll be able to plan the trip to the hospital with ease.

Things to do with Preggo No. 5

Set up a wind turbine on Her side of the bed. Don't let all those nocturnal emissions go to waste. My wife could have powered a small city towards the end of the pregnancy.

Chapter Five

Strippers, Midwives and Cops

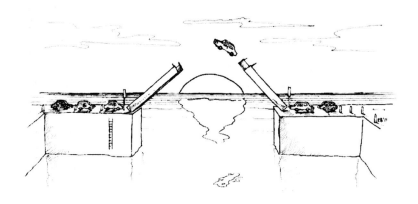

"Don't worry Love. We'll be at the hospital before you know it."

Oh my God it's coming out!

You are never fully prepared for the moment she goes into labour. Just accept it, man up and start moving. This is the moment you've trained for soldier. You are going to be scared shitless and ready to run screaming for the hills but remember that however scared you are She is a million times more so and with a million times greater reason too. This is your time to step up to the plate and be a man. We've all heard the expression anyone can make a baby but it takes a man to be a father. Never a truer group of words spoken but that's not all. You need to be a man from now on.

Don't wait for the kid to come out. Now is your time to be there for her: completely and utterly. This is the scariest thing she has ever done and there is no backing out for her. Whatever happens, She has to deliver this baby. She is going to experience pain the likes of which you have never experienced. Imagine every kick in the nuts you've ever had. Now imagine all that pain added together, multiplied by fifty and you aren't even close. Now imagine that pain lasting for hours. Now imagine you are experiencing that pain naked from the waist down for all that time while strangers walk by and occasionally peer up your ass. I'm barely touching the surface here but you get the idea. This is going to hurt and she knows it. She's more scared than she's ever been so you have to be her rock. It doesn't matter what you're feeling - bury it.

You're a man, you've bottled up everything else in your life so suck this up and be strong for her. I used to joke in my act that my feet were killing me during labour but could I get any sympathy? Guys loved that bit. Women, not so much. Try and distract her. Puppet shows are good. Rating the hotness of the midwives is not. Tell her over and over how proud you are of her and that she's going to be an excellent mother. Unlike men, women think about hundreds of different things at the same time and at this moment in their lives they are inundated with every insecurity imaginable:
- Will I be a good mother?
- Will the baby be okay?
- What if I don't love it?
- What if it doesn't love me?
- Will I get my figure back?

- Will he still find me sexy after this?
- What if I poo myself?

You need to help allay as much of this as possible.
- Of course you will.
- Of course it will.
- Of course you will.
- Of course it will.
- Of course you will.
- Of course I will.
- I will fall about laughing and keep reminding you about it at family get togethers.

You have to allow for the last one. I said be a man, not a wuss. Anything to do with poo or farts is funny. No room for discussion. It just is.

Stevie's month by month guide to the creature inside her: 8th month

It's getting so big now that it doesn't have much room so it won't be kicking as much and merely wriggles around. Freaky fact: it now has regular sleeping times and can even dream. Can't imagine they'd be that interesting though.

In the delivery room while my wife was giving birth there was an incredibly comfy looking leather armchair placed lovingly in a corner. I say comfy looking because I wasn't dumb enough to try to sit in it.

It's a trap!

Stay away from the chair. If you dare plonk your testosterone filled ass on that chair for even a second you will unleash the combined fury of one agonised woman and at least six overworked, underpaid female staff and the resulting carnage will make the movie 300 look like Finding Nemo. That chair is a test. Just like her asking if her bum looks big or if you think her best friend is hot, it's a test. Men only have to fail one of these tests once to endeavour to never fail another. As you peer around her gigantic arse trying to get a glimpse of her hot best friend you will lie more convincingly than Bill Clinton when faced with semen stained dress and a soggy cigar. Forget the chair exists. It only leads to pain.

Why does no-one care what I think?

Because you're a man. End of story.

You may have helped to put the baby there but let's face it, there's bugger all you can do to get it out.

The Drive of your Life.

We've all seen the movies where the screaming woman is driven through the streets at breakneck speed screaming obscenities with the driver encouraging her to breathe while he simultaneously screams obscenities at every other driver on the road. In the vast majority of cases this probably won't happen. That is of course unless you drive like that all the time and your wife is a sailor.

There is a chance that she will go into labour while She's at work or out shopping or while you're away and if that's the case you're just going to have to wing it. Most women however are at home when labour begins so it's a good idea to prepare as well as you can for that eventuality. Firstly, make sure that you have a route planned to get to the hospital. If you don't drive and are going to rely on public transport then make sure that you know the correct times of everything and more importantly, what time they stop running. Have the numbers of a few taxi firms in case one is busy or has gone out of business and finally have someone on standby with a car, either a friend or relative who knows to keep their phone on in case they are needed as a last resort.

If you have your own car then firstly, make sure it's in good condition; keep it full of petrol, oil etc. There is nothing more suspicious than filling up at a petrol station in the middle of the night while a woman screams in the back seat. We've all seen Silence of the Lambs. You also don't want to break down on a lonely road and end up delivering the baby yourself. Drive the route to the hospital a few times and at different times during the day. A route which might be plain sailing at night might be gridlocked during the day so have alternative routes planned. If this is your first baby you have no idea of the insanity that is the school run with hundred's of women in 4x4's who have no idea how to drive them. You would be safer driving through the dodgems at the Annual Road Rage Carnival. As with people relying on public transport, have a good knowledge of all the different ways to the hospital and have taxi numbers etc. This is one of those moments where you will get to shine and no matter how much preparation you make I promise you it won't be wasted. Anyway, you're a man. You love this type of shit. I know I did.

Top five appropriate songs to play during labour:

1. "Push it" by Salt'n'Peppa
2. "It's a mans world" by James Brown
3. "Ballcrusher" by WASP
4. "Break on through" by The Doors
5. "Love Hurts" by Nazereth

My wife was already in hospital due to a pre-eclampsia scare when she went into labour with our first child so I just hopped in a taxi at 2.00 am and let him do the swearing. My time to do the hell for leather drive came with my second son. I was literally getting into bed at 2:30 am after coming home late from a gig when my wife sat bolt upright and uttered the immortal words "I think my waters broken". I resisted the urge to use the old "Don't worry honey, I'll just pop to the kitchen and get you another", gag (BTW, So should you. Not the time, trust me). Off we went on a 3:00 am dash to cover the 20 miles to the maternity hospital. There was practically nothing on the road so I have to admit I was enjoying myself immensely save for the odd distraction of my wife moaning about something or other every now and again. I had completed around one third of the journey when I thought all my prayers and movie star fantasies had been answered. As I tore through a thirty mile an hour zone at seventy five I passed a police car.

I could see it all. They would spin around in a cloud of tyre smoke and chase me down. I would pull over and jump out to explain. They would then say follow us and it would be blue lights and sirens all the way to the hospital stopping only long enough to get the cop's name so that I could name my child after it. (In my fantasy the cop's name was cool like Rick or Thor, not Norbert or something). Well, I must have passed them on the way to a doughnut sale because they never even glanced at me. I was gutted. It ruined the whole pregnancy experience for me I must admit.

Pelvic Toning Devices

You can get barbells and vaginal weights for women to exercise their pelvic floor muscles. I'm not a woman, or a doctor but I've been to plenty of gyms and I can't see how a woman can pick up a barbell with her vagina. To be honest, I never want to meet a woman who can.

Delivering the baby yourself.

I don't mean as a money saving exercise. There is a chance, however miniscule, that for some reason the baby starts coming out and there's no one around but you. As an absolute last resort you may have to deliver the baby so it's a good idea to have an idea of what to do and most importantly, what not to do.
It really is very rare for a labour to progress so quickly that you don't have time to get to the hospital but it does happen. The good news is that; normally, if the birth is moving that fast it means that everything is going great. The bad news is that you have to step up to the plate. Well behind it anyway. (That's a baseball reference. Look it up, it's really quite clever when you understand it). Don't be too eager to jump in and help. No matter what you or her think you only need to deliver the baby if the head is showing so no dramatic cries of "Stand back, I'll deliver this baby" just because she had a touch of wind in the supermarket. If you can't see the baby and more importantly if the baby can't see you either then there's probably time to get her to the hospital or call an ambulance.

If She has a problem and no one else can help and if you can find them maybe you can hire The A-team, dah dah dah daaahh, dah dah daaahh. Sorry, forgot what I was doing there for a moment. Okay, lets assume that the baby is coming out, the A-team are nowhere in sight and you're the only thing between baby and the floor then here is a step by step guide to saving yourself years of medical training.

Firstly and most importantly don't panic. Keep as calm as possible. Remember, this is the scariest moment of her life so far and she definitely didn't envisage the drooling moron who put the baby in there to be the one who's in charge of getting it out so the calmer you are the better it is for her. Ring emergency services and then lie to her about how long they'll take to get there. Next, lay her down on top of something clean like towels, blankets, newspapers or the shirt off your back if necessary. Place something soft behind her. If you can, scrub your hands with soap and water or hand sanitizer up to the elbows. You've seen enough movies to know how to scrub up so get to it.

Encourage her to pant throughout and to push only gently with each contraction. The panting is to try to prevent tearing. If all goes well the baby's head will come out and this is when you need to be ready. Once the head is visible place your hand on it to support it and get her to push. When the head is out cradle it gently and get her to stop pushing. The baby will quarter turn to get its shoulders out and then come flying out of the vagina like a greased pig. I'm aware that isn't the nicest metaphor for the arrival of a new life but it really shoots out of there. The next step is an important one. Catch the baby, I can't stress that enough.

If the umbilical cord is not around baby's neck leave it alone. (The cord not the baby). Gently stroke downwards along the baby's nose to expel any fluid and mucous. The baby should cry at this stage but if they haven't after thirty seconds give its feet a wee slap and if this doesn't work you can try blowing gently into its mouth. This should cause the baby to cry and you can then place the baby onto Her chest and encourage her to try to breastfeed the baby as this helps with the body's expulsion of the placenta. Leave the umbilical cord and the placenta attached to the baby and sit back and rehearse how well you're going to tell this story in bars across the land for many years to come. Sit back happy in the knowledge that you can end every argument with her from now on with the phrase "Who delivered your baby when no one else was there? That's right; I did so Pretty Woman is a crap movie and let that be an end to it."

I've taken great pains throughout this section to keep reminding you not to cut the umbilical cord. Not because I'm afraid that the baby will go shooting around the room like a balloon with the air coming out. (Although I truly wish they would. Imagine.) The truth is that the umbilical cord is the literal lifeline between mother and baby and any mistake with cutting it could cause the baby to bleed to death. Remember in the first Matrix movie? How tricky it was for Trinity and Morpheus to extract Neo from the Matrix? Well, let's just pretend that it's exactly like that.

All that being said however there is one instance when you would have to cut the cord. In the event that the cord is wrapped around the baby's neck and is cutting off it's air supply then you may have to cut it (The cord not the baby and if you thought of the band Air Supply when you read that last sentence go back and start this section again. Clearly, your head is not in the game).

What one piece of advice would you give to a man on how to handle his pregnant partner?

Park your rationality outside the house. You are now in a new regime. Logic is out and emotions are in. You must do the following: shower her with attention, leave her alone, bring her surprises, bring her routine, be calm, be passionate, behave and be there. You also need psychic abilities to know when to switch between all of the above. Remember it's only a phase, albeit a very long one.

Tomas, University Lecturer

If this is the case firstly get two pieces of twine, string, shoelaces etc. anything that you can tie off the cord with. Tie off the cord tightly around four and eight inches from the baby and then cut the cord in the middle of these two knots. Gently unravel the cord from around the baby and make sure the baby is breathing by going through the steps we spoke about earlier. Make sure that the knots in the cord are tight and that there is enough space between the knots and where the cord is cut so that they don't come loose as this could lead to the baby bleeding to death. If She delivers the placenta keep it safe as the hospital will want to do some tests on it.

I've outlined above what you should do to deliver a baby. Now go back and read it again. Commit it to memory. You won't have the time to riffle through this book looking for the relevant section should the unthinkable occur so bone up now. Now that that's taken care of I am going to talk about something much more important. What not to do. In his book "Emergency Birth; a Manual" Dr. Gregory White puts it beautifully. He says, "When in doubt. Do nothing."

He's absolutely right. Babies have been born in fields, caves, taxis and even occasionally hospitals. In the majority of cases nature takes over and the baby comes out just fine. Your role is to catch it when it's delivered and to keep it and her safe until the professionals arrive so don't suddenly think you're a midwife and start pissing around. Here's what not to do.

Firstly, and I'll say it again. Do not cut the cord. I saw a great movie once where a guy helps a woman give birth while around fifty guys are trying to kill them. He actually shoots the umbilical cord to cut it. Now I don't want to go putting ideas into your head. Yes it was one of the coolest things I've ever seen but just don't. I've told you the only time you should cut the cord. That's it. Do not pull on the baby's head to coax it out or pull on the chord. I won't go into the fairly obvious reasons why. Just don't. That's pretty much it. The odds are you'll never be in this position but if you do end up delivering a baby at the roadside remember to be modest, tell the press that she did all the work and you'll look like an even bigger hero. Most importantly of all though. Make sure to tell them where you learned how to do it and also where others can buy this helpful and let's face it, lifesaving book.

What happens when we arrive at the hospital?

After what may or may not be a hell for leather dash to the hospital she will waddle up to reception where she will be sat in a wheel chair and brought into the pre- labour ward where she will be examined, poked, prodded and generally violated while the medical team assesses how far along in the labour process she is.

The Perineum

The perineum is the area of muscle between the woman's vagina and anus. Or the chin rest as it is known in some circles.

If she is more than seven centimetres dilated she will be brought to the labour ward and the party starts. If, on the other hand, her contractions are still quite far apart and she is not dilated then she will be moved into a ward where the waiting begins. This can go on for a very long time which is boring as hell for you, and also for her except her boredom is punctuated with bouts of excruciating cramps and abject terror. Walking her up and down the hospital corridor (It is known as The Green Mile in the Rotunda Hospital in Dublin. Proof positive that women are tough, making jokes at a time like that. Legend).

This can be a good time to get something to eat for both of you. It helps keep your blood sugar up and it may be the last time she will feel like eating for ages. Also use this time to make sure you have paid up your parking if necessary. She will not appreciate if during the last stage of labour you pop out to avoid getting a ticket. (Selfish of her I know but there you go.) As I say, this can go on for a long time, hours and hours. Both of you should try to conserve your energy because you will need it later - you especially. She will be a bit too busy to sleep when the pushing starts and maybe even a little bit sore too (snigger) and you'd be amazed how pissy she would get if she watched you snooze in the corner during this time. Eventually, after many examinations she will be declared dilated enough to have the baby and it's off to the labour ward. Then the real fun begins...

What are the three stages of labour?

Well, there's the main stage, the indie stage and the dance tent. Oh, sorry, that's a music festival. Labour has been divided up

into three stages and knowing which stage she's at is very important. The three stages of labour are known as;
1. The First Stage.
2. The Second Stage.
3. The Third Stage.

How dull and unimaginative is that? Let's come up with our own names. From now on the three stages of labour shall be known as;
1. The cervix opens like a flower at dawn stage.
2. Time to shove a coconut right through that flower stage.
3. Wait for the rest of the coconut plant to come out too stage.

Poetic and descriptive I think you'll agree. I don't see them changing all the medical textbooks just yet but give it time.

How did you react on learning that you were going to be a father?

Having spent the previous decade celebrating every time a pregnancy test showed a negative result, it felt strange to be celebrating a positive one.

Eoin, Writer & Businessman

Simply put. The first stage is when she is having contractions which actually do something (As opposed to Braxton Hicks). During this time the cervix is opening like a yawning chasm. When the cervix is ten centimetres dilated then we move on to the second stage. This is where the actual pushing and screaming begins and doesn't end until the baby comes out. The third and final stage of labour is where the placenta and the rest of the umbilical cord come out. More and more couples are now taking the placenta home and eating it as it is a spectacular source of protein. I've included a recipe for placenta at the back of the book.

Oh God, I can't believe you looked. I was kidding. Not about the freaks who eat it, about the recipe. You thought about it didn't you? You and Hannibal Lecter.

Let's put all that unpleasantness behind us. What you want to do with your wife's organs is up to you. I'm not here to judge. Fuck it, I have to judge here. I've tried to be pretty tolerant of individualism here but can we draw the line at eating placenta? Have a protein shake. Make it with breast milk if you want to be weird. Personally I think there are only two normal(ish) options for dealing with the placenta. You can either take it home, dig a hole in your garden and plant a tree on it or you can let the hospital dispose of it.

Personally, I was happy to let the hospital incinerate it although come to think of it if I'd let my wife cook the placenta it would have been incinerated anyway (Badoom tish). If you are of a gardening bent and wish to plant a tree on it I can only offer this one piece of advice. Make sure you dig the hole deep enough. So deep that a cat can't come and dig it up. Whatever about a mouse on your doorstep but an organ?

So, there you have it. The three stages of labour explained thoroughly and professionally. Let's face it. She is the only one who really needs to know the physiological aspects of these stages (well, her and the midwife I suppose) all you need to know is that eating a piece of your woman, however temporary that part is, is wrong.

Labour, the final frontier:

Nothing I can say can prepare you for the whole labour experience. Sure, I've shown you what to bring with you and the best way to be prepared for the journey to the hospital but nothing can prepare you for the maelstrom (it means big storm) of emotions you will experience. From panic to wonder, from revulsion to boredom, (yes, there can be long periods of nothing in the early stages) every man's experience is different.

As I've mentioned before I was next to useless during the birth of my first child but having said that it doesn't mean that I wasn't on an emotional Teacups ride (I'm scared of roller-coasters). I experienced, in no particular order, fear, boredom, disgust, fascination, helplessness, arousal (weird thing…from different rooms I could hear women moaning which sounded identical to sexy moaning. I didn't have an erection or anything but at times it was a bit like being in the middle of an orgy. Until the pushing and pooping started.), anger (I always get angry when I feel helpless, you probably do too) and more fear. You may have noticed that apart from fascination there are no positive emotions listed there. That's because there weren't any. For the birth of my second son I could list elation, joy, relief, pride and many more positive emotions because I was so much better prepared both practically and emotionally.

What advice do you have to offer on being a father?

Being a Father is absolutely great – cherish the time you have. Make time. Dump the TV. Dump your eccentric hobbies for a while. Lose the job on the oil rig. Make whatever time you have with your baby, quality time – premium time! You'll never regret it.

Tomas, University Lecturer.

Thanks to me you're definitely better prepared than I was on the practical issues and this should relax you enough to be more emotionally ready. However long the labour lasts, whether its two hours or twenty two, you will experience levels of emotion you've never thought existed. I've spoken before about the many ways you can react on the birth of your child but watching Her in pain, the stress of helplessness and the physical exhaustion are going to leave you pretty vulnerable. Add to that the fact that no one, and I mean no one, in the hospital will care one iota for your feelings or discomfort makes this a pretty lonely time for you. You're just going to have to suck it up and deal with it later. There will be a later, hopefully with a glass of something potent in your hand and a stripper on your lap. (I'm joking about the strippers. I know I've said it a lot but it's probably in poor taste to start off your journey into fatherhood with some pneumatically enhanced siren grinding against your thigh. Unless of course you are stranded on a desert island with some strippers and the only way to start a signal fire is to rub your legs with strippers until a flame appears. No one would judge you for that. They forgave those people on the plane crash in the Andes for eating each other. Surely this is minor in comparison. On a side note do not eat each other except in dire emergency and yes I mean eat in the sexy sense).

I mentioned exhaustion there. You will put yourself through one hell of a workout during the labour. You will spend most of the time on your feet (unlike the lazybones lounging around in the bed) which is tiring enough but you may also have to hold her leg in the air or cradle her in a more supportive position for hours and heaven help you if you complain. Can you imagine the reaction if you were to voice your discomfort while She's screaming? The phrase "testicles for earmuffs" springs to mind. Make sure you eat discreetly and often. Energy drinks and chocolate will keep you going. I don't however recommend you sit there with a pizza while She pushes. Whatever happens and however long it takes you will get through it. You will be amazed at the reserves of energy and the ability to block out pain you have during this time. No one is ever going to congratulate you on your pain handling abilities when She has just gone through labour but you'll know.

Sod it. Here you are: "Well done man. You are a horse, you really are. I don't know how you did it. Have you got tiger DNA or something?"

There, that's your lot matey so enjoy it while you can. Now hoist that huge leg in the air and shut up. Seriously though, you'll be no use to her if you have a blood sugar crash at the worst possible moment so keep yourself fuelled and while no one will notice your efforts, you'll know. You'll know that you were a man and coped. Coped alone and stoically. (I'm not really sure what stoic means but they always seem to use it to describe real men in books. Why not look it up Steve? I hear you cry. There isn't time damn it. There's a baby being born. Get back to work.) This is one of the many thankless moments for the dad to be but you can take great pride in having done it.

Trust in the professionals but stay alert and be aware of what She and the baby are going through at all times. It was only by the observation of a Spanish student nurse that the difficulties my first son was going through in the womb were noticed and an emergency caesarean performed. She noticed that his heartbeat dropped with each contraction, something which had gone un-noticed by the other professionals. Sometimes experience makes you complacent - something which you can't be accused of. If you notice something that gives you even the slightest cause for concern, speak up. Which would you rather? Looking like a bit of an idiot in front of a roomful of people you'll never see again or realising that you could have prevented something horrific from happening. Exactly, so keep an eye on everything around you and speak up loud and clear if you need to. You're already a father even if the baby isn't out yet. Act like one.

With any luck the labour will go great. She will accept whatever drugs the hospital has to offer and the whole labour will float by on a dreamy narcotic cloud in a matter of minutes. The baby will shoot out like a greased pig. Immediately afterwards Her vagina will snap back to it's former glory with a sound like a guitar string breaking. She will then thank you for being such a supportive and helpful man while your newborn will stare up at you with an expression that seems to say "Don't worry, I'll be sleeping through each night like a drunken student and I'll only ever cry when your football team loses". You will then be treated to admiring looks from all the staff as you stroll off out into the world ready to celebrate your new formed family.

Sorry, did I say "with any luck"? What I meant to say was there isn't a cakes chance at a Weightwatchers meeting of the labour being easy. While she will be the one in agony don't for a second think that it will be easy for you either. The woman you love is going to be in the worst pain of Her life (worse than anal I'm guessing) and there is very little you can do about it. This helplessness is horrible believe me. Now, it's not so horrible that I would ever change places. Let's not spread on the bullshit here. There wasn't one second of my wife's pregnancies where I wanted to change places even if I could. After watching the labour you will mentally drop to your knees and thank the Lord that you were born without a uterus.

The labour, as we well know will be incredibly hard for Her but as I said its going to be equally hard for you. Okay, maybe not equally but still probably the hardest thing you've ever experienced. Except maybe those unwanted erections you'd get in class when you were a teenager just before you were called up to the blackboard. In the end my fervent wish for you is that you leave the hospital with your head held high, happy in the knowledge that you were there for Her, completely and utterly and even if you never receive acknowledgement for it you'll take huge pride in knowing that you are a father now and as it turns out, you have been since She told you She was pregnant.

What is your most powerful pregnancy memory?

"I used to sing and talk to the bump pretty much every day. The song I'll always sang was Dyno blow your horn – you know...I've been working on the railroad, all the live long day.... Also, I remember the first three months being hard, in terms of not being able to tell anyone – I know it's the done thing in many other parts of the world, but we wanted to keep it quiet until we got the first scan out of the way."

Daragh, Radio Presenter

Chapter Six

Pethidine and Poop

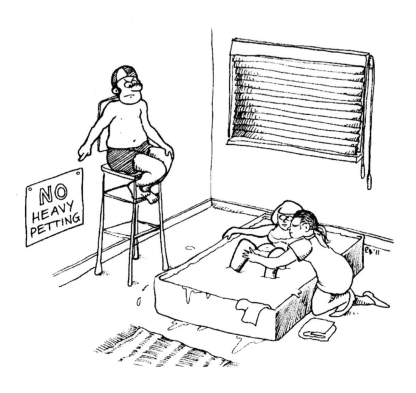

What are the most common forms of pain relief?

Apparently giving birth can be a little uncomfortable for the woman. They may have the odd niggling little twinge every once in awhile after labour has begun and some of the less hardy types may want a bit of pain relief. Well good news ladies. Not being men you aren't as tough as we are but the nice scientists have gone to all the trouble of coming up with ways to make your owies all better.

Okay, get a pen and scribble out that last paragraph. If any woman ever reads that I'll be wearing my testicles as a hat for the rest of my short, pain filled life. I can't know for sure the pain of childbirth but having witnessed someone experience it, I know one thing. I never want to. If you ever bothered to look up what a woman actually goes through during labour, the contraction of places you never knew existed etc, you would probably throw the book away and run screaming to the pub for solace. Actually, let's pretend you did look it up and go to the pub anyway. Now, don't you feel better? This pregnancy thing is a breeze.

Stevie's month by month guide to the creature inside her: 9th month

Hurrah, the baby is about to arrive or, Holy Shit, it's coming. It's pretty much squashed in there and hopefully upside down and waiting to dive on out. Freaky fact: the umbilical cord is over two feet long. Technically, if she gave birth standing up it could bungee jump

Serious time again: there are many forms of pain relief out there. Some more effective than others and some have an effect on the baby. Whatever pain relief She elects to have is her business. You have absolutely no right to stick your oar in here. If you want to dictate the pain relief by all means go ahead but you have to promise one thing first. For the entire labour you must have a six year old walk up and kick you in the testicles every two or three minutes. I'm betting that after the second kick you'll be banging heroin into yourself. (Or at the very least you'll have killed that kid.) She's the only one experiencing this pain so she's the only one who gets to decide her pain relief. You can

113

offer an opinion by all means but don't be a dick if she doesn't agree with you. Once again, her body, her rules.

The most common forms of pain relief are as follows:
- Gas and air.
- Pethidine.
- TENS machine.
- Epidural.
- Massage.

Gas and air is just that. It's a huge canister beside the bed with an oxygen mask attached. It contains a 50/50 mixture of oxygen and Nitrous Oxide (laughing gas to you and I). She can breathe deeply of it whenever the urge takes her. It is very mild and does make her feel a little wasted. It may make her drowsy but some women like the feeling while others feel a loss of control. By all means have a wee sniff yourself. Once mind you. You're no good to anyone if you're running around the corridors with a sheet around your neck, giggling like a maniac and shouting "I'm Batman, I'll deliver your baby ma'am". On second thought do it. I dare you. Think of the number of YouTube hits you'll get.

Pethidine is a narcotic. All narcotics will pass through the placenta and into the baby's blood stream. The later in labour the drug is given dictates the amount in the baby's bloodstream after birth. The disadvantages of this form of pain relief to the baby are the fact that the baby may be drowsy and therefore find it difficult to breastfeed initially. Narcotics can also depress the baby's respiration. Having said this, thousands of healthy babies are born every day with this form of pain relief but it's important to know the risks. Some women find using narcotics makes them dizzy and can cause quite severe nausea even leading to vomiting spells. I am aware that I keep using the term narcotics and it puts you in mind of every cop show you've ever seen but that's what they're called. If I called it giggle medicine you'd accuse me of not taking things seriously.

TENS stands for "Transcutaneous Electrical Nerve Stimulation". Sounds like a cross between an implement of torture and a sex toy doesn't it? In actual fact it uses an electrical current to block pain impulses while stimulating the body into producing endorphins. Four self adhesive pads are placed on either side of the spine and this is connected to a box which she can use to control the level and frequency of stimulation. (More and more like a sex toy every minute). I would recommend hiring one a couple of weeks before the due date and then you practice putting it on for her. Give her a few goes so she knows what to expect. Place a pad on your arm and feel the contraction of your muscles. It's a weird feeling but fun too. Resist the urge to stick it on to your willie. I don't know what would happen but it can't be anything good. The reason I recommend hiring one is that the hospital may not have them or they may be in use when she needs them. This form of pain relief does not affect the baby apart from maybe giving it a cool spiky hairdo.

Inarguably the most effective form of pain relief is an epidural. This is where a catheter is placed into the lower spine and anaesthesia is administered directly into the spinal cord. This causes instant pain relief and does not affect the baby in any way. I have witnessed the relief on a woman's face once the epidural is completed. It's amazing to watch. They go from agonised misery to asking for a cuppa in a split second.

The final form of pain relief I want to mention is one that you can provide. No, I don't mean going and getting something from that dodgy looking guy who hangs out in your local bar having loads of really short conversations with anxious looking people. I'm talking about massage. Around 90% of women experience back pain on top of everything else during labour. Massage from you can help to greatly relieve that. Simply massage her lower back in a gentle circular motion. This can help relax the muscles and ease the pressure that the baby's head may be placing on her Sacrum.

Freaky Fact:

Babies masturbate in utero.
Eeeeeewwwwwwwww!!!!!!!!!!!!!!!

Some women wish to give birth with no pain relief whatsoever. These women are called nutters. Well, in my opinion they should be called nutters. If I was the one giving birth I would have started taking pain relief around ten minutes after the conception and by the time labour rolled around you could hit me with a 2x4 and I wouldn't even blink. Some women want to feel everything associated with the birth and if that's what she wants then that's totally her choice. One note of caution however: once everything kicks off she may suddenly change her mind and want all the pain relief the hospital has to offer. This can cause two problems. The first being that she may have left it too late. She may suddenly decide that she wants an epidural but the labour may be too far advanced for that or the anaesthetist may be indisposed. I can imagine no greater horror than to have struggled bravely without pain relief and then to realise that you can't go on without it only to be told that it's too late. My point is, check with her frequently and reassure her that it's no failure on her part if she elects to have pain relief.

The second thing to consider is what effect changing her mind about pain relief may have on her. She may view it as some form of failure or at the very least she will be disappointed that the birthing experience was not what she planned. As I said already, reassure her that she's doing great and that there is no shame in asking for help. I would recommend a good discussion beforehand about why she wants to forego any pain relief. Is it that she's worried about what effect it may have on the baby or her own body? It may be that she is being pressured by the Tit Nazis (You'll find out soon enough) to go au naturelle. Whatever her reasons are, explore them and get her to realise that there is always a chance that she will change her mind. Get her to accept this and reassure her that whatever she does you'll be proud of her. Remind her that labour isn't a test. She has nothing to prove and there's no reward for suffering unnecessarily. Do this right and she will be much more comfortable with whatever decision she makes.

As I mentioned earlier there are no prizes for her doing the brave soldier routine. You have no right to dictate what pain relief she uses and whatever she decides to do is perfectly right for her. Personally, I strongly encouraged my wife to have all the pain relief going. She ended up using a TENS machine and electing to have an epidural towards the end of labour. I still marvelled at the strength and courage she showed throughout the whole ordeal. It's easy to imagine that the pain is only severe during the last stages of pushing out the baby but it's important to remember that women go through wave after wave of increasingly painful contractions for hours before reaching the pushing stage. I've always said that if men gave birth it would be pain free by now. We'd never have invented the car or the television. Hell, we'd probably still be living in caves but damn it childbirth would be a breeze.

What's your most powerful pregnancy memory?

"Holding my daughter for the first time. Hands down. That's how I dropped her."

Ross, Comedian.

What happens immediately after the baby is born?

As soon as the baby comes out it is placed on Her tummy and allowed to bond and stay warm. You have never seen anything quite so ugly in your life. This misshapen wailing purple creature covered in blood, poo and gore looks like something from a low budget 80's horror movie. At any moment you expect it to leap off the table and go slithering down the corridors of the hospital looking for prey. It's about here that I feel I should warn you against excessive imagination. It's hard enough being a new dad without being convinced it's the next Chucky.

Oh sure. I've heard of many men falling apart and breaking down into tears of joy at the sight of this wee miracle. This is perfectly normal and fine. If that happens to you don't worry - If you're feeling a little emasculated after the birth drop into the strip club on the way home. That should re establish the status quo. I'm sure they probably have a new dad, two dancers for the price of one special, so sit back and bask in your new found maturity. You may not feel anything. I don't mean at the strip club but that is the main rule there I grant you. I mean at the birth of your child. I personally felt a huge sense of responsibility when I held my eldest son for the first time. I was almost overwhelmed by the realisation that it was up to me to protect this completely helpless fragile creature. There's an instant lesson in maturity. I went from essentially happy go lucky wanderings to complete responsibility in an instant. The one thing that brought me back from the brink was one of the midwives came up to me and asked if I wanted to keep the placenta. I replied "No thanks. I've already eaten" True Story. It's one of the quips I am most proud of in my life. The look on the midwife's face was priceless.

The arrival of my second son brought with it a feeling of relief that both he and my wife were fine because by then I was so used to being a dad that I realised that despite all our fears, these fragile little creatures are surprisingly rugged. I don't recommend you take them mountaineering or anything but don't panic too hard. Conversely, you need to panic a little. A little bit of panic keeps you on your toes and out of the children's hospital.

Whatever way you feel on seeing your child for the first time is completely natural. You aren't an unfeeling monster if you don't bawl like the baby itself. Neither are you Big Girl's Blouse if you cry like someone suffering from depression watching Sophie's Choice (Only if you suffered from sympathetic pregnancy you girly).

Strip clubs aside however. After a while the midwife will whisk It away to wash it and dress it. You will be expected to provide the clothes from the prepared labour bag.

"Remember the labour bag? Honestly, the one thing you're asked to do and you can't manage even that small task." I've deliberately used the woman tone just to remind you what's in store if you forget to bring something to the hospital like nappies or bodysuits or Her. She may have had some tearing or an episiotomy so will need to be stitched up. You will probably finally get to hold your new life in you big clumsy fists.

There is now one person in the world who thinks you are: brilliant, funny, kind and generally an all round Mr. Perfect and as long as you give them a little bit of your time every day and are nice to their mum they'll always think that.

Eoin, Writer & Businessman

As I mentioned earlier it doesn't matter how you react. Everyone's different but I'll bet you the price of this book that whether you're crying like the baby or offering the stone face to the world you won't be able to take your eyes off your baby. You will pore over every inch of the baby marvelling at the tiny fingers, touching the tiny flat nose and if it's a boy scoffing at the tiny penis. Come on, you hardly ever get a chance to do that in the changing room so you can be forgiven for taking the opportunity when it arises. You will of course eventually get bored but by that time She should have returned and believe me She won't. Not for one second. If She is going to breastfeed; the midwife should be in to help or if you're going to formula feed then you might get to feed It. Don't worry. You'll have to feed it eventually. I know you imagined the first meal you shared with your kid being a kebab at 2:00 am when they're eighteen but no, your first solid food with him will end up all over both of you. Exactly like a 2:00 am kebab now that I think about it. Now it's time for you to bow out quietly and then go get a drink. It doesn't matter what time it is there's always somewhere open. Even if you don't drink go get a drink. Go get a drink and raise it to yourself because congratulations. You're a father. Let the games begin...

You're shitting me.

You've heard of it. She's heard of it. We've all heard of it but no one wants to talk about it. The muscles She will be using to push are the same ones she uses to poo. When the baby is coming out it is pressing directly on her rectum and practically shoots the stuff out. There is a better than fair chance that it will happen to her so here are Stevie's do's and don'ts of accidental pooping.(nice ring to that if you'll pardon the pun).

- Do try to distract Her by getting her to focus on you. She probably will not have noticed and the midwife will take care of it discreetly.
- Do not shout "There she blows" while waving your hands in the air.
- Do tell her that you are so proud of Her and that She is doing great.
- Do not point at said mess and say "It really is true. You can't digest sweetcorn"
- Do resolve to never speak of the incident and allow Her the bliss of ignorance of this embarrassment.
- Do not edit the labour video with the 1812 Overture as a soundtrack syncing the cannon to her own explosion.

Since seeing the baby come out of Her I'm freaked out

No shit dude. Let's not gild the lily here. There is nothing beautiful about seeing a scrunched up face come stretching out of a woman's party zone. Here is a place which had, to you, only one function: to give pleasure. Oh, I'm sure women have other uses for it but I don't know and quite frankly I don't want to know. To see this lovely neat thing suddenly gaping with a person looking out is of course a shock. It doesn't make you a wimp or a bastard to feel that. Now what does make you a bastard is if you say it to her. Here's my simple advice. The same advice I'd give you if you told me that your grandmother was prone to wandering about with her dressing gown open...... Just don't look.

In fact stay away from it altogether. There's no reason for you to be anywhere near it. You're not delivering the baby so just stay up near her head offering encouraging words. She needs you up there anyway so it's a good excuse.

Human nature being what it is there is a good chance you'll have to look at some stage. (Cue image of under granny's robe). That's okay, you may not even be freaked out but there is a better than fair chance you will. If you do catch a peek there is one cardinal rule. Never tell Her. She'll ask but just say that you were too focused on her to notice. She will be freaked out at the thought of you seeing her like that. She'll worry that you won't be able to find her attractive after that so its best if she believes you never saw a thing. Time for the light at the end of the tunnel.

Worst case scenario. You saw everything. I don't know. One eye peering out at you. Whatever particular horrific scenario you choose. You saw the horror but the good news is that the next time you look everything will be back to normal. Just like if the CIA came in on some covert operation to search your home. They'll ransack the place but put everything back just where you left it and by the time you get home it's like no one was ever in there. So, there you have it. To sum up. Try to avoid looking down there. If you do look and are freaked out fear not. The fanny you know and love will be back soon. The only issue here is you. Can you get over what you've seen? Simple answer is yes. Your dick couldn't care less if he saw the entire cast of Les Miserables marching out of there. Neither should you.

Dress for success

When it comes to leaving the hospital to bring your new one home you are a complete contradiction. You are torn between the massive excitement of finally bringing this little creature you have been waiting for forever home to an almost paralysing fear as you realise you are now one hundred percent responsible for this helpless creature and you have absolutely no idea what you are doing.

Don't despair, that fear you are experiencing is well known to every parent who ever lived. When it comes to your first chid we are all clueless. Just try to feed it when it cries and try not to drop it and trust me, you'll be okay. What I am most concerned with at the moment is the outfit you will be wearing for the trip home. Your beloved will be wearing something loose and concealing which allows her to do the saddle sore cowboy walk with some modicum of dignity. The baby will be better dressed than you have ever been so that just leaves you.

Please be aware that this may well be the last time you walk anywhere without your child or at least without some badge of parenthood such as a bit of vomit on your shoulder or poop on your lap for a long time.

Stevie's month by month guide to the creature inside her: 10th month

Yeah, it can happen. Some babies take their time. Don't worry; it'll come out when it's hungry.

As I was leaving hospital with my first son I passed a new dad who was unmistakeable due to his slightly dazed and incredibly proud expression on his face. What made it hilarious was his "Who's The Daddy?" t-shirt. I'm sure he didn't realise and maybe it's just me but doesn't that make it look as though there is some doubt as to whom the father of this child actually is? I'm sure in his head as he was doing his uber proud, John Travolta, Saturday Night Fever walk through the hospital he could hear the macho tough inner voice going, "Who' the Daddy? I'm the

Daddy, Oh Yeah" whereas in actuality it looked like he was on his way to the Jerry Springer show for a paternity test.

I managed to buy a wee t-shirt for our second baby which I was not allowed to ever put on him, not least for our trip home from the hospital. My wife thought it was in terribly poor taste but I thought it was a scream. It was a simple blue t-shirt with three little words on it. Mind you they were incredibly offensive despite how hilariously cool they were. Okay, I'll tell you but this is one to keep away from the missus. It simply said…"They Shake Me"

I know, I know, but, come on, that's funny. Maybe not to most but I still laugh when I think of it. I also tried to get her to put it on him for his six week check up and his christening but no joy. Probably for the best though. I'm barred from the church as it is. Just an incident with diluted blackcurrant drink and the holy water font. How was I to know that people would think it was actually the blood of Christ and start a vigil?

My reason for telling you this about your outfit is so that you realise that you are out of the loop when it comes to dressing your baby and I think you know what would happen if you suggested clothes for your wife so you are the only one left. Dress well today because from now on you're going to look like shite……Literally.

CHAPTER SEVEN

TIT NAZIS AND TEARS

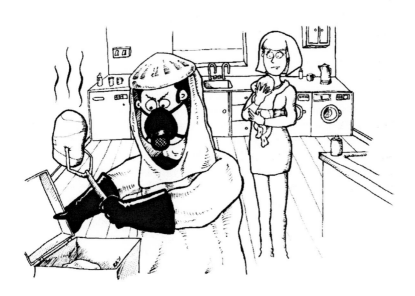

"Nothing human made that."

She won't stop crying and she wants to kill me.

Okay, this is perfectly normal. She has been a raging bag of hormones for the last 40 weeks and now that the baby is out all those hormones have to work their way out of her system. Add to that the fact that she's in pain and has been through the single most physically demanding time of her life. The important thing is to make sure that this is just the baby blues and not something more serious like Post-Natal Depression.

The baby blues are a completely common reaction to the stress and hormonal maelstrom that She has been experiencing. It manifests itself in the first few days after the birth and only lasts a short time. Symptoms of baby blues include. Weepiness, fatigue, irritability, vulnerability and mood swings. So, a normal day at the office then. Treat the baby blues as you would if she was premenstrual – with kid gloves.

It doesn't matter how irrational her behaviour is. Cut her some slack. She's wrecked: both physically and emotionally. She's just given birth and she's a woman. By that I mean her anxiety levels and worries have gone into overdrive. You have probably worried about two things. How will I be able to afford this baby and what if I'm a bad father? She has worried about:

- What if the baby hates her?
- What if she hates the baby?
- What if she makes a mistake and the baby dies.
- What if she doesn't get her figure back?
- What if He (meaning you) saw her down there?
- What if He never finds her attractive again?
- What if there's something wrong with the baby.
- The current global economic climate
- The situation in the Middle East.
- Whether her bloated pregnancy feet will ever fit into expensive strappy shoes again.

This is barely scratching the surface here. Basically the baby blues suck. Cut her as much slack as you can. Just love her and be strong and it should all be over in a few days or at most weeks. Take note of some of her more memorable and funny psychotic episodes and remind her of them later - preferably in company. I said be nice, I never said be perfect.

A much more serious situation is Post Natal Depression. This is something that you have to keep a close watch out for. You will be in the best position to notice if she's suffering and PND is not something to be taken lightly. It can start as baby blues and escalate from there. It affects around fifteen percent of women and can last for months or even years if not treated. The earlier it is recognised, diagnosed and treated the better so once again it's up to you to keep a close eye on Her.

As with so much in life the jury is still out on the exact causes of Post Natal Depression. There are a number of contributing factors which may account for some if not all of it.

Firstly if the birth was traumatic or if there was risk of injury to either the woman or the baby. The birth experience may not have been what the woman was expecting. I know to you this is ridiculous but remember women begin planning their wedding at age two. They are creatures of expectation and if something is markedly different it can affect them.

Stressful life events such as a bereavement or moving house can also be contributing factors. There are of course biological factors. Problems with the Thyroid Gland can lead to depression and let's face it She has been nothing but a maelstrom of hormones for months now. Listen up dude: an unsupportive partner can be a factor. You must remember that there has been a huge life change experienced by both of you. Her more so. She's lost her freedom and her body and if you start being a prick then she's lost you too. I know the first few months are hard for you but they can be a nightmare for her. You've done great so far. Keep it up a little while longer. If you do a good job she probably won't even notice how supportive you've been. Promise yourself a Harley Davidson when you're forty. Or an affair. Okay, maybe just the bike then.

Seriously though. Be there for her as much as you can. You will adapt to all these new changes and so will she. I promise you'll come out the other side happier and so much stronger from it.

Another potential cause of Post Natal Depression is the good old media. The image of the new mother in the media is preposterous. Some spotlessly clean, well rested, slim super model breezes around a bright spacious show house while a picture perfect baby coos up at her and waits patiently until mum has arranged her next coffee morning.

Bollocks! What they don't show you is that off camera the baby's real mother is sitting on a chair in a stained tracksuit passed out asleep while between takes the super model snorts down lines of cocaine to keep that dreamy look on her face. For all women there are days when the baby behaves and they get a chance to gussy and make themselves feel human again. There are also days where she has streaks of baby formula and shit in her hair. She's wearing a tracksuit that would have looked baggy when she was eight months pregnant and her hair hasn't seen a brush since the conception. That's a normal mother but the media will never portray that. It's little wonder that women are affected by this form of bullshit pressure.

As I said earlier it is most common for family members to notice that She is suffering from Post Natal Depression so its important that you know what to watch out for.

Symptoms of Post Natal Depression:
- Irritability.
- Anxiety.
- Fear of being left alone with the baby.
- Lack of interest in meeting friends or going out.
- Panic Attacks.
- Obsessive behaviour such as cleaning meticulously or obsessively fearing death.
- Tiredness.
- Sleep problems. Either too much or too little.
- Loss of libido.
- Loss of appetite.
- Tearfulness.

If She is exhibiting some or more of these symptoms then contact your local health nurse, your GP or the hospital. Don't assume it's nothing and don't assume it'll go away on its own. The good news is that it's completely treatable and as with most illnesses the earlier you diagnose and start treatment the easier it will be to cure.

Just because you've passed the ball off to the professionals doesn't mean your work is done. There are a number of things you can and need to do to help.

How can I help with Post Natal Depression?
- Listen. Let her vocalise all her fears and anxieties. You know women love to talk and it really helps so just let her get it off her chest.
- Take the baby off her hands as much as possible so she can rest.
- Do more housework.
- Organise times for her to go out with her friends and family so she realises that her life is not over.
- Be fun. Make her laugh. Just try to be cheerful and supportive.
- Good food. If you are a good cook, fill her up with healthy tasty food. Good nutrition is vital for both physical and mental health and it will show her how much you care,
- Love her. Even more than usual. She really needs it.

If you add your support to the counselling and perhaps medication she may be prescribed then she should make a full and rapid recovery.

There is one more condition you need to be aware of and this is called Puerperal Psychosis. It is the rarest and most extreme form of Post Natal Depression. It effects around one in every five hundred women. This usually manifests itself soon after birth with the mother exhibiting signs of confusion or psychosis. This form is usually treated with hospital care. As with the other two: with correct diagnosis, love and care She will make a full recovery.

Don't for one minute underestimate how hard this will be on you and taking care of yourself is equally important. While I have spent much of this book, and rightly so, talking about how hard it can be for her, don't worry brother, I haven't forgotten you. Let's get the niceties out of the way first. Being a father is just great. The joy your children will give you is something you can't imagine. Okay. Now that's out of the way lets get on to the cold hard truth.

It's not going to be easy. This whole thing. You've probably begun to realise since the moment you found out. She has already changed. Not just physically but in almost every way. If you were the sort of couple who loved to go out and get hammered at the weekend that's over for now. Maybe forever. Once She realises that She's pregnant She has to change her lifestyle immediately. She doesn't even get to get hammered one last time to celebrate. If she smokes she now has to stop. No discussion here really. There's no doubt that it's bad for the baby so if She wants to do well by her child she has to stop. I know that's really preachy but it's a fact. I know many people who say that their mother smoked and it didn't do them any harm. Maybe the fact you're defending something so stupid gives credence to the fact that you might be a lot smarter if your mother had quit. Some women expect their partners to quit smoking alongside them in solidarity. Speaking as an ex smoker, screw that. Give up smoking for your health by all means. Better yet, do it so that you may live longer to be a father to your child but if you are coerced into quitting like that it's unlikely to work and you'll only resent Her for asking you. Now, you'd better stop smoking in the house or anywhere near Her though. It's the least you can do.

Back to how shit it is. Let's go through some perfectly common thoughts and feelings that you could never voice to her. Not your mates, or your family. Maybe to a barman but that's it.

It won't stop crying and I want to kill it (The baby).

Babies cry. It's their only means of communication - literally. Babies cry when they're hungry, sad, scared, lonely, tired, have a wet nappy, have a dirty nappy or have an unfashionable nappy. Okay, that last one, not so much, but you get the picture. Your baby will cry, sometimes for what seems like days at a time and yes you will have homicidal urges towards it. This does not make you a monster (unless you act on it obviously) and you are not alone. Apparently a baby's cry can reach higher decibels than a pneumatic drill.

Imagine a builder using a pneumatic drill at the end of your bed at three in the morning. Now, imagine that the only way to stop him was by wiping his arse and feeding him a litre of milk from a bottle. Not a pretty image I grant you. Now imagine having to do that every three or four hours for months. Wouldn't you cheerfully strangle that builder? Of course you would. Just because it's your child making the racket does not make it any easier to put up with. There are an astonishing amount of weird folksy remedies to get a baby to stop crying. The internet is full of them and it can't hurt for you to have a look. I believe that the reason there are so many is because every baby is different and diff'rent strokes for diff'rent folks as they say.

Whatchoo talkin' bout Steve?

Sorry, that reference is a wee nostalgia trip for anyone over the age of thirty five. But, I digress. Check out all the techniques on the internet by all means and believe me there will be no shortage of parents with their own sure fire sob stopper. The simple fact of the matter is that you will come up with your own that works for your baby. You will manage it but it may take a while so you need to prepare for the worst case scenario.

Which is?

The Demon baby. The Demon baby is not a myth. I've seen it. It can scream at full volume, without getting tired, for hours and then start all over again after a few minutes sleep. It seems to have an instinct for knowing the precise second you enter deep sleep and then counts to five and off it goes again. Sleep deprivation is one of the most effective forms of torture and is in fact banned by The Geneva Convention. Captured enemy soldiers are protected from it but parents aren't. That would be funny as hell if you weren't so tired. Rest assured, the Demon Baby is incredibly rare, as rare in fact as the Angelic Baby.

The Angelic Baby is a joy to behold. They sit happily playing with their toes when not being bathed or fed and greet you with a smile after sleeping soundly for twelve hours. They don't crap. They produce rose scented pellets which come out already wrapped in a nappy bag. They are, in a word, perfect. Most babies fall somewhere between the two. Sometimes they cry, sometimes they coo and you can rarely predict when. As I once again labour the point here are my tips for surviving the crying:

Take turns. There's no point in you both being exhausted. Be honest with each other and whomever is closest to cracking should get out of the house for twenty minutes. That gives them time to get their head back together and whoever is stuck with the enemy knows that they too have a break coming. Check your child. Check to see if your child has a physical problem. Are they hungry? Do they need a nappy change? Are they in pain? If the answers to these are no then put the baby safely in its cot and walk out of the room. Even five minutes can save your sanity.

Get help. There are a number of excellent phone lines you can use who are brilliant at calming you down if you are ready to crack. Once again, put the baby in a safe place and ring them up. Just talking to someone who understands and won't judge you can work wonders. Try a change of environment. Take the baby for a drive in the car or for a walk in the buggy. Even if this won't get the little horror to sleep it can save you from that feeling that the walls are closing in.

If the worst comes to the worst, leave home. Just walk out. The rule is you're not allowed to take anything with you. Not your car keys, bank card nothing. Just the clothes you stand up in. Well, you've just abandoned a woman with a small baby. You didn't think it was going to be easy do you? Once you get to the bottom of the road and start missing your TV, turn around, head back home and gain some solace in the knowledge that like Maximus Decimus Meridius in the movie Gladiator. You shall have your vengeance in this life or the next...

Top five names you should not call you son because of rhymes:

1. Luke - Puke
2. Bart - Fart
3. Andy - Randy
4. Billie - Willie
5. Buckface - .....well you get the idea.

The First Bath.

Without doubt the first truly terrifying moment for me with my first son was the first time we gave him a bath. We had been given a brief, and in my opinion half-assed, description of the correct way to bath a baby which as you can imagine went in one ear and out the other as all directions do on entering the male brain. So now, there I was holding the most fragile, important and slippery creature on the planet and was somehow supposed to wash him without dropping, drowning or traumatising him for life. I was genuinely pouring with sweat like a bomb disposal expert with the hiccups after just a few seconds of dipping him into the bath, brimming with approximately half an inch of water. By the end I had used one entire roll of cotton wool and had practically flooded the house but I had a clean baby. A clean baby who then took the biggest shit of his young life in the bath. I thought "Sod it" and lifted him out, towelled him off and ignored the faint reek of poop coming off him. Fatherhood at its finest I think you'll agree.

Fast forward to the first bath of my second son and I was like a flair barman making cocktails for supermodels. I was flipping my son around like a rag doll secure in all the knowledge that I had acquired from bathing my first son. Namely, babies aren't as fragile as we think and with experience comes confidence. Simply put, you will be equally terrified but as with all things baby, the more you do it the easier it becomes. Or, you could always drive your hands into burning coals and then pretend that your injuries are an allergic reaction to baby shampoo. Extreme I'll admit but effective. A final word of warning however; No more tears is an advertising slogan not a guarantee. The odds are the baby will scream the house down for the first few baths. My advice here is to make soothing whale noises. Better yet, why not join a whaling ship and then you can return when all this baby nonsense is over. I think that I've just accidentally discovered the parental equivalent to Monopoly's Get out of jail free card. Simply join a whaling fleet and harpoon your troubles away. Sod Greenpeace.

I don't think Her body will go back to the way it was:

Well, you're right. It won't go back to the way it was. For example, her nipples will have darkened during pregnancy and that won't change back. She'll probably have some cellulite, her breasts will be less firm, her hips will have widened and if she doesn't do her pelvic floor exercises then her vagina won't be as tight.

That's life dude. Let's get some perspective here. I want you to place a large mirror on the floor and lean it against the wall. Next I want you to take off all your clothes and lie on the ground in front of the mirror. Next, I want you to open your legs and bring your knees up to your chest. Now, look in the mirror. Scarred for life huh? You're not exactly a centrefold yourself. Suddenly She looks pretty good now doesn't She?

Pelvic Floor Exercises

To some, the pelvic floor is something you buy in IKEA. To others it's a dance from the Rocky Horror Picture Show. In actual fact they're the muscles that both sexes have which aid continence and sexual function. And you thought it was just women.

Okay, I get your concerns and this particular one is a doozy. Of course you don't want her body to change. You fell in love with this woman not some dark nippled, bow-legged one. Just accept that there will be some changes to her body. It's not as though pregnancy is easy you know. Have you not been paying attention? I knew that I never should have put colouring in the back.

As I say, there will be some changes but between you, you can minimize these. After giving birth a woman is beyond exhausted. The preceding forty weeks, followed by the trauma of labour and then the constant demands of a newborn have effectively wiped her out and the last thing on her mind is getting back into shape. The tricky part is that the sooner she starts the easier it will be.

Now, you try telling her that. There's the great dilemma. If you tell her directly to do her pelvic floor exercises and encourage her to hit the gym you will be viewed as an abusive monster and in a small way they would be right. Forget kid gloves. To do this properly requires the finesse of a brain surgeon. You need to somehow encourage a return to the old body without touching the wrong nerve and watching her go off like a nuclear missile. Below is a list of subtle statements you can drop casually into conversation that should subliminally encourage her back to the old body.

1. I heard that Angelina Jolie can pick up a claw hammer with her pelvic floor. Amazing considering all the time she spends on charity work. Some women are amazing.
2. I heard George Clooney has just joined our local gym. You know the one with the unisex sauna.
3. I heard all the girls in your old school have really let themselves go. Isn't your school reunion in a few months?
4. I heard all the girls in your old school do triathlons now. Isn't your school reunion in a few months?

You can add your own to this list at any time. Be imaginative but for the love of God be subtle. Not like pushing against her head when she's resting it on your chest in the hope of a blowjob. I mean finesse.

Stevie's month by month guide to the creature inside her: 11th month

Just kidding. This almost never happens. Seriously, she would be as big as a hatchback if there was a kid still in there.

It is a genuine problem though. There will be changes to her body and the quicker she addresses them the easier it will be for her in the long run. However, telling her this is tantamount to domestic abuse. Even your friends will judge you for it. Ideally a mature open talk with plenty of reassurance that you'll always love her no matter what she looks like but for her health and well being you think she shou.........

See what I mean. I'm only talking to you and I'm shitting myself. I suppose the talk is one option but I wish you luck with it. By the way, if you're out of shape and take little or no care of your appearance then you've no right to give out to her. In my opinion, the best way forward is for you to join a gym and start going regularly. Rave on about how great it is to have some time away from the baby and how good it's making you feel. You know She can never stand to see you enjoying yourself without her so she's bound to start going. Another more effective but infinitely more sneaky way is to start going to the gym and when you get home casually mention the nice chat you had with this young woman on the exercise bike next to you. Don't oversell it. Remember be subtle. Guaranteed, she'll be packing a gear bag within minutes.

Beware the Tit Nazis

The term Tit Nazi is one I coined myself after the birth of our first child. I suddenly noticed these harridans coming out of the woodwork to pass comment on and judge everything my wife did about our newborn. These bitches (and I use that term deliberately) seem to believe that they are the all knowing baby and pregnancy experts whose omnipotence allows them to cajole and at times downright bully new mothers into doing things their way. I use the term Tit Nazi because they are usually militant breast feeders who think giving your baby formula is tantamount to putting the Ebola virus in a bottle.

Don't get me wrong. I am fully aware that breast is best and all that but bottle runs a damn close second. There is always a chance that She won't be able to breast feed or she may choose not to. It may not be conducive to your lifestyle or for myriad reasons it may not be possible. It does not make her a monster if She doesn't breast feed or if She elects to try a mixture of breast and bottle. One of my boys was breast fed while the other wasn't. They are both strong, healthy brutes who both love their mother unconditionally. The argument that bottle feeding somehow lessens the bond between mother and baby is bollocks. Pure and simple.

You must remember that a new mother is an incredibly vulnerable creature. She is exhausted, maybe still in pain, she has no confidence in her ability to look after the baby and is probably desperate for some helpful advice. That's when she is in greatest danger from the Tit Nazis. They come in the guise of helpful, experienced mothers but genuinely helping is not their priority. They want to wax lyrical about their only area of interest. Namely baby minding. They want to control and browbeat her to somehow validate their own existence. Below is a list of the traits common to all Tit Nazis;
- They do not work. Tit Nazis do nothing all day except hover around their children.

- Their husband's are visiting prostitutes. (Okay, I'm guessing here)
- They hang out in packs.
- They eat all the time. I think the grazing helps with milk production.
- They are parents to the dumbest looking, wimpiest kids you've ever seen. Blame genetics here.
- They keep shooting out babies until their husband kills himself or their womb falls out.
- They breastfeed their kids until they head off to college.

These are the women who will fill your beloved's head with all manner of horror stories. They will one up every birth story they hear. Their labour was the most difficult in history and they will terrify her with graphic stories of pregnancy nightmares. Given the slightest chance they will try to convert her to their way of thinking like some weird cult. They will have comprehensive advice on everything from feeding to bathing, from weaning to wanking. Well, maybe not wanking. Lets face it that's your area of expertise and no one would ever doubt that.

In short, these women are toxic and it's up to you to watch out for and ultimately protect her from them. As I mentioned, She is very vulnerable before and after birth so it's up to you to be her big strong protector. You have my list above to help you recognise these harpies so if you think your beloved is being affected here's what you need to do to get rid of them.
- Splash them with baby formula. This has much the same effect as holy water does on vampires.
- Tell them there's a buy one get one free offer on doughnuts and watch them waddle off at speed.
- Show them their husband's credit card bill with all the mystery brothel charges.
- Shoot them in the face with a 12 gauge shotgun. (Okay, maybe a little extreme but you'll be tempted, believe me.)

In all seriousness though. There are women out there with so little going on in their lives that they have to bring others down. If your partner comes in contact with them help her to recognise them for what they are and you never know. She may even load the shotgun for you.

What if the worst should happen?

Miscarriage.

This is going to be the only section of the book that I will not be making fun of for obvious reasons.

Around one in every five pregnancies ends in miscarriage which is a shockingly high percentage when you first hear it. While we all may have someone close to us whose had a miscarriage we don't hear about others very often. The reason for that is because of its very horror and the devastation it causes to the woman it is rarely spoken about directly. Miscarriage is a silent spectre hanging over the heads of many pregnant women. They are acutely aware of its existence but naturally don't want to dwell on it. Should the worst occur it is devastating for you both and even more so for her. I won't dwell on it and neither should you. There are enough fears surrounding pregnancy and childbirth already without focusing on the ones you have little or no control over. Miscarriages are common but not often talked about because the pain is too great. Should the worst occur there are some great supports available to you both. There are many wonderful support websites that help you realise that you're not alone and that others are surviving and hurting too. Counselling is really important for both of you also. I mentioned that she will feel this more than you and I'm afraid that's true. She will have all of the disappointment you have along with guilt, fear that she will never have a baby and countless other feelings. This is when you need to be there for her completely. Give her time, space, love and most importantly encourage her to talk. Some day you will hopefully be ready to try again and the figures show that the majority of women go on to have healthy babies after one or more miscarriages. The point is simply that despite how devastating miscarriages are there is always hope.

S.I.D.S.

Fear was my constant companion for the first couple of years of both my boy's lives. Every time they went to sleep I worried that they wouldn't wake up again. It's amazing. I am optimistic to the point that I don't have a pension plan or savings because I am definitely going to win the lottery. I cheerfully believe that everything will turn out for the best but from the moment my first son was born I was accompanied everywhere by this impending sense of doom.

S.I.D.S. (Sudden Infant Death Syndrome) or cot death as it is also known is something every parent worries about. You lie there at night straining your ears towards the baby monitor hoping the baby will snore or fart or at least breathe loudly. You lie there and convince yourself that your baby is dead so you jump out of bed and race out to check the baby only to find the object of your terrified musings lying with it's ass in the air dreaming of boobs or whatever. That's only going to happen another five or six thousand times before your child outgrows the risk and you start to breathe easy again. Every parent goes through this because we all know of someone who went through the unthinkable. People who went to their baby's cot only to find that the worst had happened. Even childless people seem to empathise because we can all imagine how horrific that must be. S.I.D.S. is real so just for your information, I won't say to set your mind at ease because nothing will but the incidences of S.I.D.S. are relatively rare. The rate is around two in every thousand babies which is reassuringly low. This rate has fallen dramatically over the last decades because of the realisation that having babies sleeping on their backs greatly reduces the risk of S.I.D.S.

The death of a child is probably the most devastating thing which can happen to a couple. I cannot imagine how hard it must be to get through something that painful. All I do know is that you have to be there for each other more than ever before. Bereavement counselling is also essential.

I've only mentioned two of the many fears you may have in this section. I'm sure you've thought of many more. Birth defects, psychological problems, etc. I have only dealt with two areas here and both really briefly. The reason for this is twofold. Firstly, I meant for this to be primarily a funny book as that's something I feel qualified to do. I am good at seeing the funny side of life and making jokes about it. Obviously there is no funny side to these fears and I do not feel even remotely qualified to write about them with the sensitivity and care they deserve.

The second reason I am neglecting to write about these fears is because it hurts to do so. Writing about miscarriage and S.I.D.S.

has made me remember the fear I went through while my wife was pregnant and while my sons were babies. It's also stirring up the fears I have for my family today. That's what it means to be a dad. You worry about your children because you love them so much. If you allowed yourself you'd imagine a million different scenarios where your child could get hurt or killed. But thankfully you don't allow yourself. If you did your life would be a paranoid hell. That is the attitude you need to adopt throughout this pregnancy. Of course there is a chance that the unthinkable could happen but it's just that, a chance. Be aware of them but don't dwell on them. The odds are on your side so concentrate on the positive and making this pregnancy a positive experience for you both with an amazing gift at the end. Yes, something bad may happen but if it does, you'll deal with it. You know you will.

CHAPTER 8

BLUE BALLS AND BENNY HILL

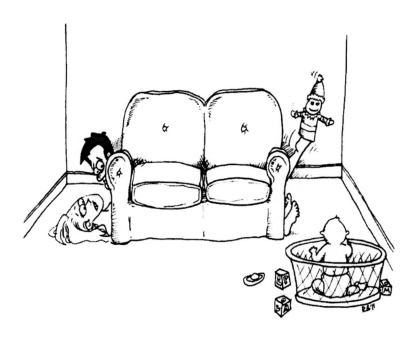

How Soon Can We Get Back to Doing the Nasty?

Let's face it. You have been through a lean spell of late. You may have not wanted to. She may not have wanted to. The baby may not have wanted you to (who wants all that knocking when you're trying to sleep?). Whatever the reason you are naturally concerned about when you can get back in the saddle so to speak.

Okay, the science bit. After the birth a woman's vagina is in bits. I read one description that said giving birth is like a small explosion going off in her vagina. (How cool would it be to do one of those, slow motion, back-to-the-explosion walks like in action movies just after the birth?) As with any explosion there's always going to be some collateral damage and she needs time to heal so even with a straightforward birth you need to wait until after her six week check up. If she's had a tear, episiotomy or caesarean birth it may take longer. She may be tender for much longer than that so leave it up to her and for God's sake be patient. Remember all those body insecurities and exhaustion etc.

Give her time, as much as she needs. You've been through dry spells before. Now, you don't have to be non-sexual. Clitoral stimulation is fine for her and there's no risk to her if she orgasms so go find out where the clitoris is and have fun. She can obviously help you by taking matters into her own hands if you get my drift. She can also take matters in mouth. Two options which I'm sure you'll agree are not to be sneezed at (unless that's your thing. I'm not here to judge you.) Do not perform oral sex on her as there's a risk of infection and an even greater risk that you may actually blow air in there by accident and that can be fatal – seriously! So, wait until she gets the all clear and then wait until she gives you the all clear and remember for the first time, go easy she may still be a bit tender. Don't forget the squirty boobs risk too.

As I've said earlier its sometime after six weeks when sexy time can begin again properly. Don't be freaked out if you're not jumping right back into the saddle straight away. Okay, we've mentioned it twice. I might also ask why you use a saddle in bed but hey. I'm not here to judge you. Freak.

What I'm saying is, don't go setting an alarm for six a.m. on the morning of the sixth week and jump up expecting some goodies. There are a number of factors which may hold either of you back. I mentioned the aftermath of Her fanny bomb but there are other things to consider. She may still be sore. She may be turned off by her body. She may be too tired. She may be suffering from Post-Natal Depression. She may have had a caesarean and isn't fully healed yet. She may have a baby hanging off her boob or a million other reasons. (Okay, a million reasons is a bit excessive. If She can come up with a million reasons not to sleep with you, you're fucked. Or more accurately you're not and probably never will be again.) Alternatively, you may be too tired. You may be turned off by her body. You might still be a bit freaked out by the memory of the labour. You may be looking at your willie thinking that he got you in this mess once and you don't trust him anymore. You may not be fully healed yet (from all the self-love over the past few months. Calluses anyone?).

In other words don't be worried if you don't get back doing the nasty for quite a while. Don't for one second underestimate the strains a baby puts on your sex life. The exhaustion is a major factor for both of you. I mentioned earlier that if the two of you were offered eight uninterrupted hours in bed you'd sleep, not shag. Don't underestimate the effect that tiredness has on both your libidos. I know you've probably had lazy, sleepy sex before where you languidly yet sensually move together until a gentle drifting off post orgasm. That was a few years ago and the tiredness was due to an especially late return from a party. This tiredness is as a result of ten months of pregnancy for Her and the last couple of months being under the yoke of the world's most demanding tyrant for you both.

Tiredness of course isn't the only factor. You may not find Her body attractive anymore and this is a horrible feeling. The woman you love doesn't turn you on anymore and you're torn apart by the rightfully selfish thought that your sexlife is going to be internet based from now on. On top of that the guilt you'll feel for not finding the woman you love attractive.

You love Her, She's the mother of your child, you're going to spend the rest of your lives together and you don't find Her attractive anymore. Most men experience this to some degree.

Especially after the birth of their first child because they don't know what to expect. There is also the change in how you view Her. You now see Her as a mother and let's face it, no one want to sleep with their mother (I'm talking to you Oedipus).

The whole situation is a nightmare. It's also extremely common and the great news is, it's not permanent. I believe it makes you both better lovers because you learn to focus 100% on what you're doing and the fact that it is so rare and fragile makes it quite mind blowing at times. But before we get into that we need to be aware of Her.

It's not all rosy in the garden for Her either. She will still be carrying pregnancy weight and six weeks simply isn't enough time for her to recover fully. She will recover, but it will take time. She will get used to the changes in Her own body as time goes on too. Remember, She will be even more aware of all these changes than you are and will be feeling much worse. She will be all too aware of her body's changes and will be aware of your feelings however careful you are to hide them. This is an especially difficult thing to come to terms with. Add to that all the exhaustion, the trauma of labour and everything else that goes on in her head and you now find that neither of you are feeling especially sexy.

Fear not though my friend. I said earlier that it's not permanent. It isn't. What you're both feeling is incredibly common even if most people are too embarrassed to talk about it. Take your time and allow you both to get used to the routine of having a baby and to get used to whatever body changes you both have undergone (I'm looking at you Mr. Comfort Eater when I'm tired or horny). As I say, you will get back in the saddle and believe me, the sex will be better than ever.

Why?

One word: quickies.

When you both start finding each other sexy again you will find that only half the battle has been won. You are now no longer at war with your own minds. You now have that wee tyrant to contend with. Babies have an innate ability to know when a man is around a minute from orgasm and choose that time to wake up and demand access to the boobs you just happen to be holding. They choose one minute from eruption because it's close enough to be painful to stop but long enough away that you can't convince Her to wait sixty seconds and let you finish. Selfish of both of them I know. I never really understood the expression Blue Balls until I had a child. Making up a bottle feed while your testicles twist around each other is not something I'd recommend. The risk of your manhood getting trapped in the bars of the cot is also a consideration. (Come on, no it isn't. Have you seen how wide the bars are? I could rattle mine along it like a tin cup in a prison movie).

But Steve, I hear you cry with the slightly higher register that comes with Blue Balls, you said that sex would be better than ever. I did and it will. Because of the fleeting nature of your sex life you'll find that you both get really good at giving and taking pleasure fast. I mean fast. Not just you.

I'm sure that if there was a sexual sprint competition you'd be world champion but She also learns to take it when She can get it. No more half an hour of foreplay for her. It's a case of Wham Bam Thank You Sir in this case. This selfishness teaches you both how to get maximum pleasure from each other for minimal time. Baby falls asleep in the living room, mummy and daddy race for a knee trembler in the downstairs toilet. Baby falls asleep in the car daddy begs for a blowjob. Baby falls asleep in the shopping trolley; mummy and daddy go and violate the frozen food section.

Because sex has now become this almost forbidden fruit (Stay out of the fruit and veg section, it's unhygienic. At least everything in frozen foods is wrapped. Show some consideration for other shoppers) it adds a new thrill to it all. That and the fact that it could end at any second makes it doubly desirable. For an added thrill I find listening to the old Benny Hill Show theme tune really matches the rhythm of the act. Wear headphones though, She probably wont appreciate the humour.

So, there you have it. Despite what may be a rocky restart to your sex life you will have sex again and if you can avoid getting arrested for public decency offences it will be better, more fulfilling and shorter than ever.

Will we ever go out again?

Yes you will....eventually. Of course, you'll start off small. To begin with you'll hire a babysitter and hide in the garden shed with a baby monitor just to make sure everything's okay. After a few evenings like this you may even bring down a couple of packets of crisps. After all it is your night out. Treat yourself.

After your child turns seventeen or eighteen you might be up for a trip to the cinema. See, it's not all doom and gloom. Obviously, I'm being facetious. Of course you'll get out. You'll even get drunk and you will definitely enjoy those drinks or that movie more than you ever dreamed possible. It is, however, unbelievably hard the first time you go out after the baby is born. You could leave the baby with a team of paediatricians, Dr. Miriam Stoppard and Jesus and you'd still worry. And however much you're worrying, multiply it by fifty and you have Her. Mama bears, Lionesses, Mama Walton. All ferocious when it comes to their young. Thanks to the maternal instinct (Don't worry, there is a paternal instinct. See what happens when your kid is two and another two year old slaps him. I've had to be pulled away from some toddlers), She is hardwired to believe that her child needs her twenty four-seven and to leave her baby in the hands of a stranger is tantamount to child neglect. All you can do is, take her out and help her to forget that she's a mum for a few hours. This is usually best done by the administration of copious amounts of cocktails. As usual though, you need to decide who's on duty when you get back and who, more importantly, is getting up in the morning. A good rule of thumb is, if this is your first night out after the birth then let her have most of the fun.

If she is breastfeeding and cannot or does not want to express then you get to be the drunken slob. Whichever one of you is the booze hound, the sober one cannot hold it against the drunk one and no banging of pots and pans the following morning. If she is the one drinking there's a good chance that these are the first drinks she's had in months. Let her go a little nuts if she wants. She's earned it. You are bound to have wet the baby's head quite a number of times before she came home from the hospital. In fact you probably saturated the damn thing. Either way, as with all matters baby: think baby steps.

One thing that's important to bear in mind is that She hasn't been drinking properly for over a year and so is far from match fit. She will try to drink as much and as fast as She used to and believe me She'll pay for that. I have lost count of the number of women I've seen heading out for their first night with the gals since the baby was born only to return home two hours later paralytic. They made the mistake of drinking like someone who'd been out the previous weekend not someone whose liver is as shiny as a bald guys head in August. The same thing happens to submariners and prisoners. So, baby steps and no tequila shots for the first night. If she's just given birth and also just finished a two year stretch for stealing a submarine its best that she doesn't drink at all.

What advice do you have to add on being a father?

Don't think of it as 'Game Over'. If you do it right you've just progressed to a bonus round of the same game. Parents who let the baby's routine dictate everything and stop doing all the things they used to do, end up with no life. Whereas, if you get the baby to fit in with your existing lifestyle, your life just got a billion times better. (Terms & conditions apply and having a carrycot perched on the bar in your local at midnight isn't "getting the baby to fit in").

Eoin, Writer & Businessman

You may well be the type of couple who are able to plonk their baby at the grandparents and fly off to Paris for the weekend. If you are, more power to you. If you are like the majority however, start off small. A trip to the cinema or a meal out in the local restaurant is a good starter (if you'll pardon the pun). Soon you'll realise that there is a life to be led without baby and you'll be drunk and naked on the roof of a police car doing the Macarena in no time. You go girl.

It's really important to remember that you are not just parents; you are a couple as well. You love each other and even though you'll spend most of the night alternately talking about or worrying about baby don't forget to make time for each other. Remember to compliment each other.

"This light really brings out the bags under your eyes" or "Your hips seem to be returning to normal". Beware though, all this romantic talk could lead to a brother or sister in nine months. Fat chance of that. If you two had the chance to spend eight uninterrupted hours together in bed you'd sleep. If you were offered another eight hours immediately following the first eight you'd sleep some more.

The First Nappy

Nothing has prepared you for the first nappy. Nothing. You may have volunteered in the Black Hole of Calcutta working as a sewage technician but the first nappy's stench and appearance will send you screaming from the room with cries of "Kill it. That can't be human." The first nappy load is mostly composed of a dark foul smelling substance called Meconium. It sounds like something that could harm Superman and once you smell it you'll believe it actually could. Meconium is basically composed of all the shit your baby absorbed in the womb. It's a mixture of hair, amniotic fluid, bile, mucus, tequila. For once I'm not kidding. Meconium can be tested for the presence of alcohol if the mother drank excessively during pregnancy. In the USA and Canada a bad test result can be sent to Child Protective Services so tell her to lay off the slammers until after the baby is born. Just think of the kick baby will get from her breast milk. Kidding. If She's breastfeeding she should go easy on the booze. If she's willing to express then she can go milk herself and then head out on the town.

Nearly all medical textbooks will tell you that Meconium is in fact sterile and odourless. Bullshit. It may be sterile but I know what I smelled. I once was unfortunate enough to come across a road kill skunk. It was twenty years ago and I can still remember exactly what it smelled like. It was so stomach turning and eye watering I can still taste it whenever I think of it. I tell you it smelled like Angelia Jolie's cleavage compared to both my boys first nappies.

And the colour! It's a really dark brown, almost black, and is the texture of really thick molasses. It sticks to everything and anyone with a vivid imagination could imagine it oozing its way towards you hell bent on slithering up your leg and...

Okay, I have a vivid imagination. After a few days the Meconium is gone and the baby settles into a routine. The usually poop four times a day initially but eventually settle into a routine. They may poop immediately after eating or even during. Imagine taking a dump in the middle of a meal. I once was at an all you can eat buffet place (Which all men view as a challenge. Our goal is to put the place out of business). There were three very large ladies sitting across from me with piled plates. One woman went for a dump twice during her meal. (How did I know she was going for a dump. She loudy told the world each time.) She literally kept making room. I didn't know whether to be disgusted or hugely impressed. In the end I just made sure that I got to the chicken wings before her.

Let's talk about what sort of smell you can expect once the baby settles into a routine. The smell varies. Some nappies have a little dollop of vague smelling poop which can be whisked away without too much trauma. Others however, and these most commonly occur at the worst possible moment, literally cause you to gag. Your eyes will water

The only thing I can suggest is to do whatever you can to avoid changing the baby. If you walk into the room and notice that telltale waft, walk out again as if you forgot something important. Join the army and get stationed abroad if necessary. You may think that last is a little severe but you haven't smelled it yet. For our second baby my wife and I came up with the rule that whoever was holding the shitty baby had to change it. Being a man I spotted a huge loophole in that contract. I would say something guaranteed to tug at her uterus like "Oh, He wants his Mama", hold out the baby and her delight would ensure she didn't notice the smell until I had safely passed off the creature. I would then skip away while she had to go delving into the murky depths. Sure it nearly led to divorce but that was a small price to pay.

The only thing that smells worse than your own kid's nappies is other people's kid's nappies. You could have two kids on identical baby formulas and the one that's not yours smells ten times worse. They are also more stupid, uglier and more likely to end up in prison.

My quick list of things that you can do which temporarily make things easier but in the long run come back to bite you in the ass.

This is a tiny list for after the baby is born. It's a couple of quick words of advice which may help to save your sanity in the long term. There are many others but I'm planning on writing another book about raising small children so consider this a free taste. Kind of like when a drug dealer gives you a free bag just to get you hooked.

Taking the baby into the bed with you:

This is a very attractive proposition in the first few months, particularly if the baby is being breast fed. The baby gets to latch on and eat to its heart's content and then drift off to sleep in its mama's arms. The positives to this are, for her, she can feed the baby and may also be able to sleep at the same time while you don't have to stir at all. This sounds like a win-win situation but believe me you'll regret it. Your baby will be very slow to settle into a routine of sleeping. It will find your bed to be the comfiest place on earth and you will be less motivated to try to establish a routine.

Giving your baby a pacifier, dodo, sucky.

Call it what you want but a pacifier is a monkey for your baby's back. It's okay to give one for the first couple of months because apparently up until three months you can discontinue its use without your baby noticing. After that it's like trying to keep a fat guy out of KFC. Continued use of a pacifier can lead to dental problems, slow speech development and even socialising difficulties. Trust me, a child who learns to suck their thumb or the corner of a blanket will be a lot happier in the long run.

GLOSSARY OF TERMS YOU WISH YOU NEVER KNEW.

Afterbirth: Also known as placental expulsion is where the placenta comes out of the birth canal after the baby is born. This time is known as the third stage of labour.

Birth canal: Get used to canals in pregnancy. There's the birth canal, the cervical canal, the conception canal (Well this is only if you knocked her up on a path beside a canal. Not unheard of)

Braxton Hicks: These are mild uterine contractions commonly known as false labour. Usually felt in the second and third trimesters. Also the name of the third album by Australian prog rock band Jebediah.

Breech: This as we all know is a part of a gun and is usually what jams when the baddie looks set to win. It also means when a baby is upside down or something. Let's just concentrate on the cool stuff. Okay if you must know it's when a baby wants to come out ass first. It's a good indicator of what it's going to be like as an adult.

Caesarean section: This is where the baby is brought into the world through the sunroof. For whatever reason the baby is delivered through surgery.

Cervical canal: It's the canal of the cervix, duh.

Cervix: There is an old gag which talks about the polite gynaecologist saying to the woman. I'm at your Cervix. In actual fact the cervix is the lower portion of the uterus where it joins with the upper end of the vagina. None the wiser huh?

Colostrum: This is the first milk produced which is chock full of antibodies and nutrients. Basically a really good welcome to the world meal for the baby.

Contractions: These are the niggling little pains which may trouble her somewhat during labour. Listen dude, if you don't know what contractions are you probably shouldn't be breeding

Epidural: This is an injection of analgesic and anaesthesia through a catheter into the spinal cord which causes instant pain relief.

Episiotomy: This is where the doctor will make a cut to widen a woman's vagina to ease the baby out and prevent tearing. Don't worry; they sew it back up afterwards. Slip the surgeon a fifty and he might throw in a couple of extra stitches.

Fallopian tubes: These are the tubes leading from her ovaries through which the egg passes before fertilization by your mighty tadpoles.

Head engaged: This is where the baby's head meets another head and they fall in love. In reality it's when the baby is finally in the correct position for birth. Think of a break-dancer spinning on his head and you're not far off. Obviously, if the baby is actually spinning you should inform the midwife.

Induction: This is when She gets given a place in the Football Hall of Fame for her achievements on the field. Hang on; it might be when the doctors elect to induce labour through drugs. This occurs if there is no sign of labour well after the due date or if there is a fear that the baby will be too large if left to grow in there any longer.

Montgomery's Tubercules: These are little raised lumps which will appear on the aureoles of her nipples which help to lubricate the breast for breastfeeding. Also handy for teaching Braille.

Mucus plug: This is a plug which forms at the entrance to the cervical canal at the beginning of pregnancy and acts as a barrier to bacteria. A few days before labour this can be discharged by the woman. It's also known as the bloody show. I always thought that True Blood was the bloody show.

Natal: This is the adjective used for all things pregnant.

Ovaries: These are where the woman gets her eggs from. Not the supermarket. Think of them as a woman's testicles. They produce an egg once a month whereas we produce millions of sperm every day. That's the battle of the sexes won I think.

Ovulation: This is the time once a month when the ovary releases an egg and she turns into a psychopath.

Pethedine: This is basically a synthetic form of morphine which dulls the pain of labour. Some women swear by it while others get sick. It does cross the placenta however so baby can get a little wasted.

Progesterone: This is the bastard hormone which causes everything from haemorrhoids to backache - the original pain in the ass.

Stretch marks: these are basically purple lines which form in the dermis layer of the skin around the seventh month when the skin is being stretched too much. They fade in colour and may be improved by creams containing vitamin E. Personally. I think that If stretch marks were caused by stretching the skin then every man's penis would look like a road map of Los Angeles.

Trimester: This is a three month period. Seriously dude, try to keep up.

Ultrasound: This is where they photograph the baby in utero. Don't expect many costume changes though.

Ventouse: This is a vacuum device which is used to help deliver the baby as an alternative to a forceps birth. It's very safe but your baby may come out with a pointy head. Ever see the movie Coneheads? Exactly like that. Don't worry, it's not permanent. Funny while it lasts though.

Vernix: or Vernix Caseoea to give it its proper term is a waxy, cheese like substance which covers the skin of some newborns. It has many functions including temperature regulation, moisturising and lubricating the skin for passage through the birth canal and also as a tasty dip for chips or crudités. Okay, that was gross even for me. Sorry.

STEVIE'S FINAL THOUGHTS

Well who would have thought it. I finished something I started. Not something I have been accused of often in my life I must admit. I think the reason I managed it this time is because I am a dad and this book is about being a dad, or at least getting ready to be one. When I became a dad I had to grow up fast. I had to stop half-assing everything in my life because I was now responsible for someone who relied on me for everything. Even to survive. Sure my wife was around in the background but that wasn't enough for me. I had to man up for the first time in my life.

Now, I didn't have some epiphany where I stood on top of a mountain and roared to the gods that I was now a man. My Road to Damascus moment did not have any touch of the dramatic.

Oh no. Not modern day twenty first century man. He has to express himself in a slightly different way. For me it was assembling flat pack furniture. A couple of years before my first son was born I bought a flat pack computer desk. It had all the bells and whistles; slidy outy keyboard thingy and everything. I took it home and assembled it. When I was finished I had 29 bits left over and one screw at the side had been hammered half in and then hammered down for security. The slidey outy keyboard thingy slid so far out that you could bring it with you when you went for a cup of tea. In short it was an abomination of a thing and one which I used for many years despite almost daily gouging my thigh with the screw and regularly dumping my keyboard onto the floor.
 A couple of weeks before my first son was born I had to venture into the arena of flat pack hell once more. This time to assemble his crib. This too was state of the art. It rocked. (I don't mean Duuude, this crib rocks man. I mean rocks, as in back and forth). It had a locking mechanism and a wooden bolt which could be adjusted to control the movement of the crib.

Does the nursery rhyme Rock-a-bye Baby ring a bell? Given my past history it seemed that the baby, cradle, mobile, baby monitor and anything else I touched was destined to come down. Come down hard. I should never have been given the responsibility of constructing the place where this helpless infant was going to spend the majority of its time. My wife playing some mad form of baby Russian Roulette whenever She decided to rock the thing. It was madness.

It was with a heavy heart that I picked up the indecipherable instructions and set to work. Four hours later I was standing, staring down at the most perfectly put together piece of furniture you've ever seen. Every nut and bolt accounted for and rocking with the silent competence of master craftsmanship. Since then I have put together cribs, cots, beds, bookcases and bicycles for my boys and each one has been perfect. The reason is simple.

When it came to my boys I did it right. I focused and concentrated. I didn't just shout Fuck It and reach for the hammer. I couldn't. I was responsible.

Two months ago I put together a bookcase for our living room. When I was finished one pane of glass on the door was cracked and the left hand side had been put on upside down which necessitates the wedging of two paperbacks under it just to keep it from falling over. It wasn't important enough for me to go back and fix it. I couldn't muster up the hyper focus I'd employed when it came to something that was designed for my boys. I swear I never consciously put extra effort into assembling my boy's stuff in the same way that I never consciously half-assed the bookcase.

In the case of my boys I just did it right and so will you. You won't have to consciously try to do what's right by your child, you'll just do it. You'll do it because that child is a part of you. Without you it wouldn't be here. You'll do it because you'll love that child more than anyone or anything. More than life. It's clichéd I know but it's also true.

I'm sure you're scared about so much that's coming down the line. I hope I've addressed some of them in this book. I didn't want you to be flippant about the whole thing but I did want you to have a laugh. Well, lots of laughs if I'm honest. My main reason for writing this book came from one source however: my wife. (Yeah, Yeah, You love your wife. That's so gay)

I said earlier that I was a real help to my wife when she was in labour with our second child. I really was. I wanted to help other men to help their partners too. (Damn it. I got through nearly the entire book without referring to Her as your partner. Shit) I hope that you've found genuinely helpful advice here that will help you to be a better man for her throughout this time. I also hope that you found enough of your own private thoughts voiced in these pages to make you realise that you're not alone. All men go through this when they are about to become a father. All men get scared. All men get angry. All men have times when they wish, however briefly, that it wasn't happening. All men get through it.

The fact that you've read this book says a lot about you. It says that you have excellent taste and a wicked sense of humour. It says that you find farts funny and that you're obsessed with boobs. It also says that you love Her and that you want to help and be there for Her. It says that you understand that you have a responsibility to Her and your unborn child and it clearly says that you're man enough for that responsibility.

Whatever you think of yourself and whatever anyone thinks of you, some day very soon you're about to become the greatest guy in the world...

You're going to be a dad. And whether you know it or not you're ready.

Also Available from Glasnevin Publishing

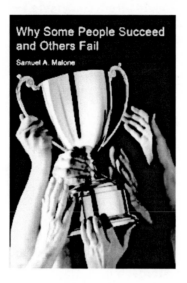

Why Some People Succeed and Others Fail
By Samuel A. Malone
2011
ISBN: 978-0-09555781-8-2

In this inspiring and remarkable book you will discover the principles of success that have directed and motivated many people to make a significant contribution and difference to the world. You will also uncover the pitfalls to avoid in your quest to become the best you can be.

Success in any endeavour does not happen by chance. It happens through the application of sound principles and purposeful actions such as: Setting realistic goals, Making worthwhile plans, Practising good interpersonal relationships, Having confidence and self-belief, Being optimistic, Developing self-esteem, Being persistent and resilient, Being highly motivated, Developing the habit of lifelong learning and continuous improvement, Practising good personal values

This book has an entertaining blend of inspirational real life stories, quotations, practical tips, acronyms and activities to help you acquire the right habits and practise the skills of success. The book is underscored by the best scientific research currently available which is made accessible to the reader through clear simple language. By following the principles set out in this book you will become the happy and successful person you are destined to be.

Samuel A Malone is a self-employed training consultant, lecturer and author. He is the author of 20 books, some of which have gone into second editions and foreign language translations.

Visit: www.glasnevinpublishing.com for more titles and information

Also Available from Glasnevin Publishing

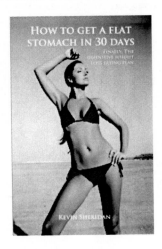

How to Get a Flat Stomach in 30 Days
By Kevin Sheridan
2011
ISBN: 978-0-09555781-9-9

You will NEVER have to go on a diet again...Are you ready to embark on the most rewarding and exciting challenge of your life? The weight loss technique shown in "How to Get a Flat Stomach in 30 Days" has proven to be virtually 100% successful for those who genuinely apply its principles. The good news is that this book gives you all of the tools to obtain a flat stomach in 30 days and keep it! You will discover the secrets that others have paid thousands to learn.

This book will show you: How to lose weight easily using the latest scientific findings. How to feel motivated and healthy, and to increase your energy levels. How to use the unique "MERC" weight loss formula. An effective 30 day program that will remove years of accumulated toxins from your body. How to identify and remove the foods and chemicals that depress your metabolism. Effective exercise techniques and programmes to remove excessive fat. Imagine, you can lose up to 15 pounds (6Kg) in 30 days... permanently! The secrets and techniques in this book will even help you to burn fat while you sleep! This book promises "your best ever shape" and you will not be disappointed, because it really works!

Kevin Sheridan is one of Ireland's leading weight loss experts. He is an NCEF qualified personal trainer with over twenty years of experience specializing in weight loss, toning and fitness. He lives and works in Dublin where he is a full time personal trainer and a frequent contributor to radio and TV programmes where he specialises in weight loss. He also lectures on college courses in fitness and health.

Visit: www.glasnevinpublishing.com for more titles and information

. Also Available from Glasnevin Publishing

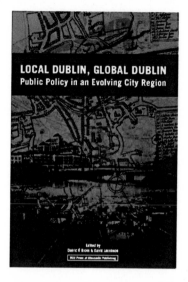

Local Dublin Global Dublin: Public Policy in an Evolving City Region
By Deiric O'Broin & David Jacobson
2010
ISBN: 978-0-09555781-4-4

This timely volume examines the state of public policy formulation in the Dublin city region and the implications for the key public policy processes and regional stakeholders of ongoing and potential changes in the region's economy and its relationship with other comparable city regions. The contributors offer elected representatives, policy makers, citizens and communities some considered advice that draws on past experience and the lessons learned from other countries. The book provides a comprehensive analysis of the key public policy choices facing the Dublin city region, including spatial planning, local development, public infrastructure, higher education, innovation, labour market intervention and sourcing international investment. Its contributors include respected economists, geographers and political scientists presenting accessible and thought-provoking analyses, and outlining a framework for public policy formulation and implementation for an evolving city region in the context of the ongoing reconfiguration of global trade and financial networks.

Visit: www.glasnevinpublishing.com for more titles and information

Also Available from Glasnevin Publishing

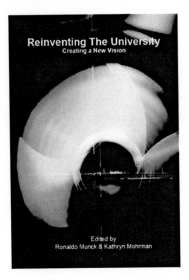

Reinventing the University
By Ronaldo Munck & Kathryn Mohrman
2010
ISBN: 978-0-09555781-5-1

"Business as usual" is no longer a viable way of running a 21st Century university. The impact of globalization, the growing complexity of the university mission and the still uncertain impact of the 2008/09 global recession all point towards a future characterised by uncertainty. Against the pessimistic scenario, however, we can discern some good reasons for optimism in regards to the university re-inventing itself for the new millennium. This book demonstrates the need for the modern university to move beyond narrow disciplinary boundaries and to become more socially embedded in order to succeed in the current competitive climate. The universities are uniquely positioned to bridge the needs of the citizen and the emerging technologies in a democratic and participatory manner. Science and technology is leaping ahead at an unprecedented pace due to globalisation, but often social needs and human ethics are not to the fore. While universities cannot retreat to an 'ivory tower' which no longer exists, they can engage with technology and the market to help make science serve social need and advance democratic citizenship in a most turbulent global era.

Visit: www.glasnevinpublishing.com for more titles and information

Also Available from Glasnevin Publishing

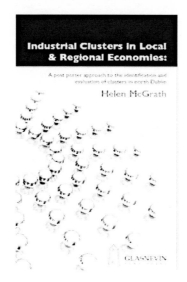

Industrial Clusters in Local & Regional Economies
By Helen McGrath
2008
ISBN: 978-0-09555781-1-3

This timely volume examines the state of public policy formulation in the Dublin city region and the implications for the key public policy processes and regional stakeholders of ongoing and potential changes in the region's economy and its relationship with other comparable city regions. The contributors offer elected representatives, policy makers, citizens and communities some considered advice that draws on past experience and the lessons learned from other countries. The book provides a comprehensive analysis of the key public policy choices facing the Dublin city region, including spatial planning, local development, public infrastructure, higher education, innovation, labour market intervention and sourcing international investment. Its contributors include respected economists, geographers and political scientists presenting accessible and thought-provoking analyses, and outlining a framework for public policy formulation and implementation for an evolving city region in the context of the ongoing reconfiguration of global trade and financial networks.

Visit: www.glasnevinpublishing.com for more titles and information

Lightning Source UK Ltd.
Milton Keynes UK
UKOW050630011211

182991UK00002B/2/P